THIS JOURNAL BELONGS TO

RUNNER'S
JOURNAL

A YEAR OF RUNNING

CHRONICLE BOOKS
SAN FRANCISCO

ISBN: 978-1-4521-2498-8

Manufactured in China

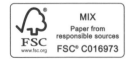

MIX
Paper from
responsible sources
FSC® C016973

Designed by Michael Morris

10 9 8 7 6 5 4 3 2 1

Chronicle Books LLC
680 Second Street
San Francisco, California 94107
www.chroniclebooks.com

About This Journal

Whether you're a casual jogger or a competitive runner who is training for races, you most likely fit your running into a busy life, which means it can be easy to lose track of goals, personal bests, the nuances of your workouts, and even simply the number of miles/kilometers you've run from week to week and month to month. We all have many ways to track ourselves in this age of quantified living, but there's something especially satisfying about writing it all down in a journal. You can fill it up, page through, reflect on what you've recorded, and, ultimately, keep and refer to it as your running evolves over time.

Use the front section of this journal to track your overall running practice over the days, weeks, and months you run. At the end of the year, you'll have created a visual summary of your year of running, annotated by you with all the details of your year's runs. Throughout the year, fill in the week-by-week sections to create a more detailed log of your weekly running.

For many of us, running began as a commitment to exercise more and has become a practice that keeps us energized through our days and punctuates our weeks. As we hustle through our daily responsibilities, running is something we do for ourselves. So is this journal. Fill it in, make lists, and, above all, use it as a tool to help you improve and enjoy your running even more.

Pre-Run Stretches

DESCRIPTION	DURATION
	TARGETED MUSCLE GROUP
	COMMENTS

DESCRIPTION	DURATION
	TARGETED MUSCLE GROUP
	COMMENTS

DESCRIPTION	DURATION
	TARGETED MUSCLE GROUP
	COMMENTS

DESCRIPTION	DURATION
	TARGETED MUSCLE GROUP
	COMMENTS

DESCRIPTION	DURATION
	TARGETED MUSCLE GROUP
	COMMENTS

DESCRIPTION	DURATION
	TARGETED MUSCLE GROUP
	COMMENTS

▶ CONTENTS

DESCRIPTION

DURATION

TARGETED MUSCLE GROUP

COMMENTS

DESCRIPTION

DURATION

TARGETED MUSCLE GROUP

COMMENTS

DESCRIPTION

DURATION

TARGETED MUSCLE GROUP

COMMENTS

DESCRIPTION

DURATION

TARGETED MUSCLE GROUP

COMMENTS

DESCRIPTION

DURATION

TARGETED MUSCLE GROUP

COMMENTS

DESCRIPTION

DURATION

TARGETED MUSCLE GROUP

COMMENTS

3 AT-A-GLANCE RECORD
Post-Run Stretches

DESCRIPTION	DURATION
	TARGETED MUSCLE GROUP
	COMMENTS

DESCRIPTION	DURATION
	TARGETED MUSCLE GROUP
	COMMENTS

DESCRIPTION	DURATION
	TARGETED MUSCLE GROUP
	COMMENTS

DESCRIPTION	DURATION
	TARGETED MUSCLE GROUP
	COMMENTS

DESCRIPTION	DURATION
	TARGETED MUSCLE GROUP
	COMMENTS

DESCRIPTION	DURATION
	TARGETED MUSCLE GROUP
	COMMENTS

DESCRIPTION	DURATION
	TARGETED MUSCLE GROUP
	COMMENTS

DESCRIPTION	DURATION
	TARGETED MUSCLE GROUP
	COMMENTS

DESCRIPTION	DURATION
	TARGETED MUSCLE GROUP
	COMMENTS

DESCRIPTION	DURATION
	TARGETED MUSCLE GROUP
	COMMENTS

DESCRIPTION	DURATION
	TARGETED MUSCLE GROUP
	COMMENTS

DESCRIPTION	DURATION
	TARGETED MUSCLE GROUP
	COMMENTS

Favorite Cross-Training

DESCRIPTION

HOW OFTEN

WHY DO IT

HOW IT FEELS

LONG-TERM RESULTS

DESCRIPTION

HOW OFTEN

WHY DO IT

HOW IT FEELS

LONG-TERM RESULTS

DESCRIPTION

HOW OFTEN

WHY DO IT

HOW IT FEELS

LONG-TERM RESULTS

DESCRIPTION

HOW OFTEN

WHY DO IT

HOW IT FEELS

LONG-TERM RESULTS

DESCRIPTION

HOW OFTEN

WHY DO IT

HOW IT FEELS

LONG-TERM RESULTS

DESCRIPTION	HOW OFTEN
	WHY DO IT
	HOW IT FEELS
	LONG-TERM RESULTS

DESCRIPTION	HOW OFTEN
	WHY DO IT
	HOW IT FEELS
	LONG-TERM RESULTS

DESCRIPTION	HOW OFTEN
	WHY DO IT
	HOW IT FEELS
	LONG-TERM RESULTS

DESCRIPTION	HOW OFTEN
	WHY DO IT
	HOW IT FEELS
	LONG-TERM RESULTS

DESCRIPTION	HOW OFTEN
	WHY DO IT
	HOW IT FEELS
	LONG-TERM RESULTS

Favorite Routes

1.

6.

2.

7.

3.

8.

4.

9.

5.

10.

Favorite Long Runs

1.

2.

3.

4.

5.

6.

7.

8.

9.

10.

Shoe Log

Depending on the shoe make and style, terrain, gait, and, of course, your own body, shoes can last for 200 to 400 miles/322 to 644 kilometers of running. Only you will know when you need to change them out or transition in a new pair. Track your shoe use here, making sure to note your comments about initial and ongoing orthotics fit and wear patterns throughout the lifespan of the shoe to help guide your decision when purchasing your next pair.

BRAND/STYLE			MILES/KILOMETERS RUN
			COMMENTS
SIZE	DATE PURCHASED	DATE RETIRED	

BRAND/STYLE			MILES/KILOMETERS RUN
			COMMENTS
SIZE	DATE PURCHASED	DATE RETIRED	

BRAND/STYLE			MILES/KILOMETERS RUN
			COMMENTS
SIZE	DATE PURCHASED	DATE RETIRED	

BRAND/STYLE			MILES/KILOMETERS RUN
			COMMENTS
SIZE	DATE PURCHASED	DATE RETIRED	

BRAND/STYLE

MILES/KILOMETERS RUN

COMMENTS

SIZE	DATE PURCHASED	DATE RETIRED

BRAND/STYLE

MILES/KILOMETERS RUN

COMMENTS

SIZE	DATE PURCHASED	DATE RETIRED

BRAND/STYLE

MILES/KILOMETERS RUN

COMMENTS

SIZE	DATE PURCHASED	DATE RETIRED

BRAND/STYLE

MILES/KILOMETERS RUN

COMMENTS

SIZE	DATE PURCHASED	DATE RETIRED

BRAND/STYLE

MILES/KILOMETERS RUN

COMMENTS

SIZE	DATE PURCHASED	DATE RETIRED

BRAND/STYLE

MILES/KILOMETERS RUN

COMMENTS

SIZE	DATE PURCHASED	DATE RETIRED

AT-A-GLANCE RECORD

One-Year Shoe Log

Color in the shoe each time you get a new pair,
so you have a visual of when and how often you
changed shoes.

MONTH _June_

1	2	3	4	5	6	7
8	9	10	11	12	13	14
15	16	17	18	19	20	21
22	23	24	25	26	27	28
29	30					

MONTH _____

MONTH _____

MONTH _____

MONTH _____

MONTH _____

MONTH _____

MONTH _____

MONTH _____

MONTH _____

MONTH _____

MONTH _____

MONTH _____

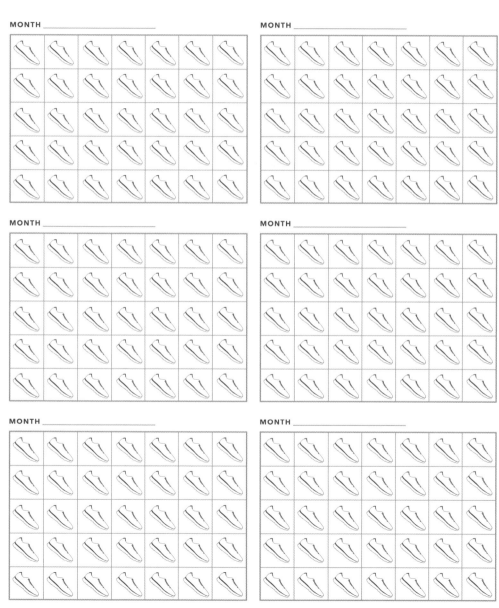

Gear to Get (or Covet)

1.) ....

2.) ....

3.) ....

4.) ....

5.) ....

6.) ....

7.) ....

8.) ....

9.) ....

10.) ....

11.) ....

12.) ....

13.) ....

14.) ....

15.) ....

16.) ....

17.) ....

18.) ....

19.) ....

20.) ....

Pre-Long Run and Race Fuel

EAT/DRINK

WHEN

EFFECTS

COMMENTS

EAT/DRINK

WHEN

EFFECTS

COMMENTS

EAT/DRINK

WHEN

EFFECTS

COMMENTS

EAT/DRINK

WHEN

EFFECTS

COMMENTS

EAT/DRINK

WHEN

EFFECTS

COMMENTS

EAT/DRINK

WHEN

EFFECTS

COMMENTS

EAT/DRINK

WHEN

EFFECTS

COMMENTS

EAT/DRINK

WHEN

EFFECTS

COMMENTS

EAT/DRINK

WHEN

EFFECTS

COMMENTS

Races to Run

RACE NAME	DISTANCE	LOCATION	DATE	RUNNING PARTNER(S)

RACE NAME	DISTANCE	LOCATION	DATE	RUNNING PARTNER(S)

Short-Term Goals

1.) ....

2.) ....

3.) ....

4.) ....

5.) ....

6.) ....

7.) ....

8.) ....

9.) ....

10.) ....

Long-Term Goals

1.) ....

2.) ....

3.) ....

4.) ....

5.) ....

6.) ....

7.) ....

8.) ....

9.) ....

10.) ....

11.) ....

12.) ....

Running Around the World

Pinpoint the cities and countries you run in as you travel for work
or play throughout the year and note the details of those runs.

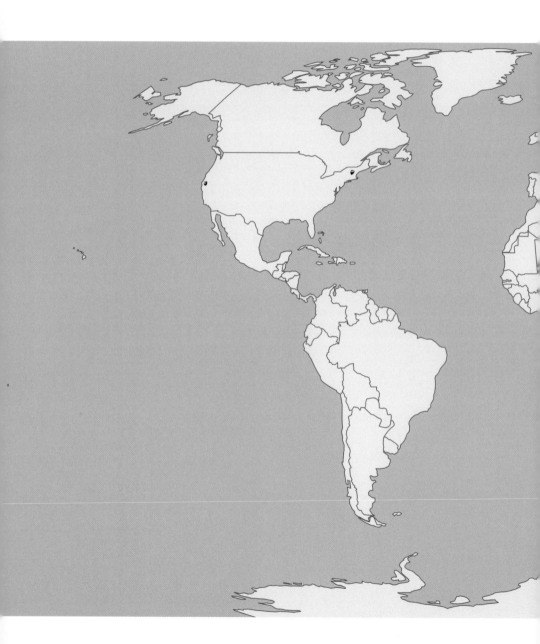

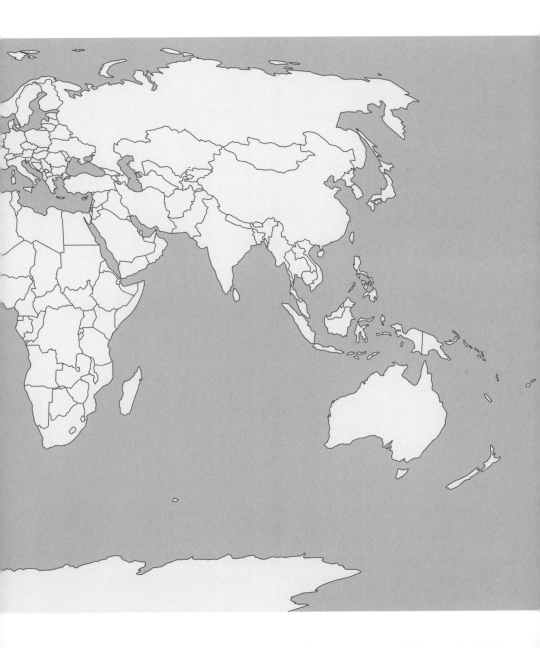

CITY/COUNTRY

RACE NAME

DATE

DISTANCE/ROUTE

NOTES

CITY/COUNTRY

RACE NAME

DATE

DISTANCE/ROUTE

NOTES

CITY/COUNTRY

RACE NAME

DATE

DISTANCE/ROUTE

NOTES

CITY/COUNTRY

RACE NAME

DATE

DISTANCE/ROUTE

NOTES

CITY/COUNTRY

RACE NAME

DATE

DISTANCE/ROUTE

NOTES

CITY/COUNTRY

RACE NAME

DATE

DISTANCE/ROUTE

NOTES

CITY/COUNTRY

RACE NAME

DATE

DISTANCE/ROUTE

NOTES

CITY/COUNTRY

RACE NAME

DATE

DISTANCE/ROUTE

NOTES

New Places to Run Bucket List

1.) ....

2.) ....

3.) ....

4.) ....

5.) ....

6.) ....

7.) ....

8.) ....

9.) ....

10.) ....

Techniques to Try

1.) ~~inline experiment 5 min pet 10 n pet~~

cd 15/16

2.) slow down new layer

3.)

4.)

5.)

6.)

7.)

8.)

9.)

10.)

AT-A-GLANCE RECORD

Symptom Tracker

Track your unexpected physical symptoms. Finding patterns and triggers will
help you prevent and manage injuries and improve your running experience.

SYMPTOM	FIRST EXPERIENCED	RECURRENCE(S)

POSSIBLE CAUSES	ACTION TAKEN	RESULTS	RESOLVED OR ONGOING?

Treatment Record

Record details of visits to health care providers and keep their contact information.

PROBLEM

HEALTH CARE PROVIDER

NAME ....

SPECIALTY ....

OFFICE ADDRESS ....

....

PHONE ....

DATE

NATURE OF EXAM

DIAGNOSIS

PRESCRIBED TREATMENT

FOLLOW-UP VISIT?   YES   NO

DATE

TAKEAWAYS

COVERED BY INSURANCE?   YES   NO

TOTAL PAID OUT OF POCKET ....

COMMENTS

PROBLEM

HEALTH CARE PROVIDER

NAME ....

SPECIALTY ....

OFFICE ADDRESS ....

....

PHONE ....

DATE

NATURE OF EXAM

DIAGNOSIS

PRESCRIBED TREATMENT

FOLLOW-UP VISIT?   YES   NO

DATE

TAKEAWAYS

COVERED BY INSURANCE?   YES   NO

TOTAL PAID OUT OF POCKET ....

COMMENTS

PROBLEM

DIAGNOSIS

HEALTH CARE PROVIDER

PRESCRIBED TREATMENT

NAME ....

SPECIALTY ....

OFFICE ADDRESS ....

....

PHONE ....

DATE

FOLLOW-UP VISIT?   YES   NO

DATE

TAKEAWAYS

COVERED BY INSURANCE?   YES   NO

TOTAL PAID OUT OF POCKET ....

NATURE OF EXAM

COMMENTS

PROBLEM

DIAGNOSIS

HEALTH CARE PROVIDER

PRESCRIBED TREATMENT

NAME ....

SPECIALTY ....

OFFICE ADDRESS ....

....

PHONE ....

DATE

FOLLOW-UP VISIT?   YES   NO

DATE

TAKEAWAYS

COVERED BY INSURANCE?   YES   NO

TOTAL PAID OUT OF POCKET ....

NATURE OF EXAM

COMMENTS

PROBLEM

DIAGNOSIS

HEALTH CARE PROVIDER

PRESCRIBED TREATMENT

NAME ....

SPECIALTY ....

OFFICE ADDRESS ....

....

PHONE ....

DATE

NATURE OF EXAM

FOLLOW-UP VISIT?   YES   NO

DATE

TAKEAWAYS

COVERED BY INSURANCE?   YES   NO

TOTAL PAID OUT OF POCKET ....

COMMENTS

PROBLEM

DIAGNOSIS

HEALTH CARE PROVIDER

PRESCRIBED TREATMENT

NAME ....

SPECIALTY ....

OFFICE ADDRESS ....

....

PHONE ....

DATE

NATURE OF EXAM

FOLLOW-UP VISIT?   YES   NO

DATE

TAKEAWAYS

COVERED BY INSURANCE?   YES   NO

TOTAL PAID OUT OF POCKET ....

COMMENTS

PROBLEM

DIAGNOSIS

HEALTH CARE PROVIDER

PRESCRIBED TREATMENT

NAME

SPECIALTY

FOLLOW-UP VISIT?   YES   NO

DATE

OFFICE ADDRESS

TAKEAWAYS

COVERED BY INSURANCE?   YES   NO

PHONE

TOTAL PAID OUT OF POCKET

DATE

NATURE OF EXAM

COMMENTS

PROBLEM

DIAGNOSIS

HEALTH CARE PROVIDER

PRESCRIBED TREATMENT

NAME

SPECIALTY

FOLLOW-UP VISIT?   YES   NO

DATE

OFFICE ADDRESS

TAKEAWAYS

COVERED BY INSURANCE?   YES   NO

PHONE

TOTAL PAID OUT OF POCKET

DATE

NATURE OF EXAM

COMMENTS

Physical Therapy Record

Note your physical therapy instructions here and keep a record of compliance.

PROBLEM	PRESCRIBED TREATMENT	PRESCRIBED FREQUENCY/ DURATION

DATE PERFORMED	DATE PERFORMED	DATE PERFORMED	DATE PERFORMED	DATE PERFORMED	DATE PERFORMED	DATE PERFORMED

Medication Record

Monitor your running-related medications to understand your patterns of use.

MEDICATION
DATE
USED FOR
DOSAGE
EFFECT

MEDICATION
DATE
USED FOR
DOSAGE
EFFECT

MEDICATION
DATE
USED FOR
DOSAGE
EFFECT

MEDICATION
DATE
USED FOR
DOSAGE
EFFECT

MEDICATION
DATE
USED FOR
DOSAGE
EFFECT

MEDICATION
DATE
USED FOR
DOSAGE
EFFECT

MEDICATION

DATE

USED FOR

DOSAGE

EFFECT

MEDICATION

DATE

USED FOR

DOSAGE

EFFECT

MEDICATION

DATE

USED FOR

DOSAGE

EFFECT

MEDICATION

DATE

USED FOR

DOSAGE

EFFECT

MEDICATION

DATE

USED FOR

DOSAGE

EFFECT

MEDICATION

DATE

USED FOR

DOSAGE

EFFECT

Races Run

RACE NAME

TIME

DISTANCE

DATE

AGE-GROUP PLACE

OVERALL PLACE

LOCATION

BIB NUMBER

DO IT AGAIN?

RUNNING PARTNER(S)

COMMENTS

RACE NAME

TIME

DISTANCE

DATE

AGE-GROUP PLACE

OVERALL PLACE

LOCATION

BIB NUMBER

DO IT AGAIN?

RUNNING PARTNER(S)

COMMENTS

RACE NAME

TIME

DISTANCE

DATE

AGE-GROUP PLACE

OVERALL PLACE

LOCATION

BIB NUMBER

DO IT AGAIN?

RUNNING PARTNER(S)

COMMENTS

RACE NAME

TIME

DISTANCE

DATE

AGE-GROUP PLACE

OVERALL PLACE

LOCATION

BIB NUMBER

DO IT AGAIN?

RUNNING PARTNER(S)

COMMENTS

RACE NAME

TIME

DISTANCE

DATE

AGE-GROUP PLACE

OVERALL PLACE

LOCATION

BIB NUMBER

DO IT AGAIN?

RUNNING PARTNER(S)

COMMENTS

RACE NAME

TIME

DISTANCE

DATE

AGE-GROUP PLACE

OVERALL PLACE

LOCATION

BIB NUMBER

DO IT AGAIN?

RUNNING PARTNER(S)

COMMENTS

RACE NAME

TIME

DISTANCE

DATE

AGE-GROUP PLACE

OVERALL PLACE

LOCATION

BIB NUMBER

DO IT AGAIN?

RUNNING PARTNER(S)

COMMENTS

RACE NAME

TIME

DISTANCE

DATE

AGE-GROUP PLACE

OVERALL PLACE

LOCATION

BIB NUMBER

DO IT AGAIN?

RUNNING PARTNER(S)

COMMENTS

RACE NAME

TIME

DISTANCE

DATE

AGE-GROUP PLACE

OVERALL PLACE

LOCATION

BIB NUMBER

DO IT AGAIN?

RUNNING PARTNER(S)

COMMENTS

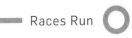

RACE NAME

TIME

DISTANCE

DATE

AGE-GROUP PLACE

OVERALL PLACE

LOCATION

BIB NUMBER

DO IT AGAIN?

RUNNING PARTNER(S)

COMMENTS

RACE NAME

TIME

DISTANCE

DATE

AGE-GROUP PLACE

OVERALL PLACE

LOCATION

BIB NUMBER

DO IT AGAIN?

RUNNING PARTNER(S)

COMMENTS

RACE NAME

TIME

DISTANCE

DATE

AGE-GROUP PLACE

OVERALL PLACE

LOCATION

BIB NUMBER

DO IT AGAIN?

RUNNING PARTNER(S)

COMMENTS

Race Times This Year

5K

RACE NAME
DATE	TIME

RACE NAME
DATE	TIME

RACE NAME
DATE	TIME

RACE NAME
DATE	TIME

RACE NAME
DATE	TIME

RACE NAME
DATE	TIME

10K

RACE NAME
DATE	TIME

RACE NAME
DATE	TIME

RACE NAME
DATE	TIME

RACE NAME
DATE	TIME

RACE NAME
DATE	TIME

RACE NAME
DATE	TIME

HALF-MARATHON

RACE NAME

DATE | TIME

RACE NAME

DATE | TIME

RACE NAME

DATE | TIME

RACE NAME

DATE | TIME

RACE NAME

DATE | TIME

RACE NAME

DATE | TIME

MARATHON

RACE NAME

DATE | TIME

RACE NAME

DATE | TIME

RACE NAME

DATE | TIME

RACE NAME

DATE | TIME

RACE NAME

DATE | TIME

RACE NAME

DATE | TIME

Longest Distances in a Single Run

DISTANCE
(MILES)

26.2 MI													
25 MI													
24 MI													
23 MI													
22 MI													
21 MI													
20 MI													
19 MI													
18 MI													
17 MI													
16 MI													
15 MI													
14 MI													
13 MI													
12 MI													
11 MI													
10 MI													
9 MI													
8 MI													
7 MI													
6 MI													
5 MI													
4 MI													
3 MI													
2 MI													
DATE													

42 KM												
40 KM												
38 KM												
36 KM												
35 KM												
34 KM												
32 KM												
30 KM												
28 KM												
26 KM												
25 KM												
24 KM												
22 KM												
20 KM												
18 KM												
16 KM												
15 KM												
14 KM												
12 KM												
10 KM												
8 KM												
6 KM												
5 KM												
4 KM												
2 KM												
DATE												

Best Times for Same Run

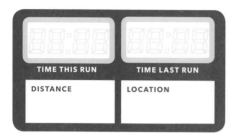

TIME THIS RUN | TIME LAST RUN
DISTANCE | LOCATION

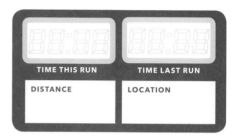

TIME THIS RUN | TIME LAST RUN
DISTANCE | LOCATION

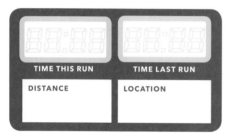

TIME THIS RUN | TIME LAST RUN
DISTANCE | LOCATION

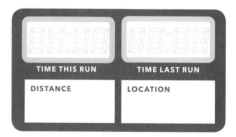

TIME THIS RUN | TIME LAST RUN
DISTANCE | LOCATION

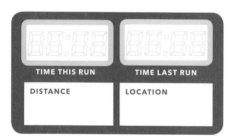

TIME THIS RUN | TIME LAST RUN
DISTANCE | LOCATION

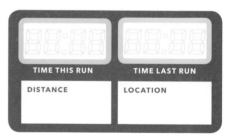

TIME THIS RUN | TIME LAST RUN
DISTANCE | LOCATION

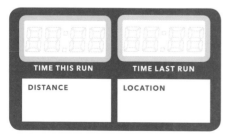

TIME THIS RUN | TIME LAST RUN
DISTANCE | LOCATION

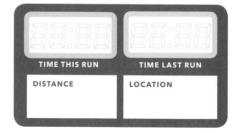

TIME THIS RUN | TIME LAST RUN
DISTANCE | LOCATION

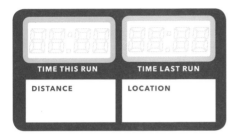

TIME THIS RUN   TIME LAST RUN

DISTANCE   LOCATION

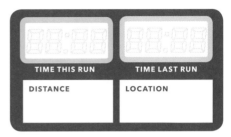

TIME THIS RUN   TIME LAST RUN

DISTANCE   LOCATION

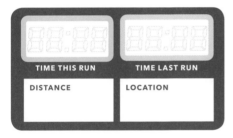

TIME THIS RUN   TIME LAST RUN

DISTANCE   LOCATION

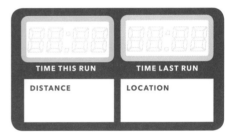

TIME THIS RUN   TIME LAST RUN

DISTANCE   LOCATION

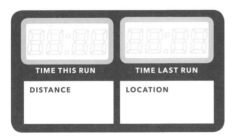

TIME THIS RUN   TIME LAST RUN

DISTANCE   LOCATION

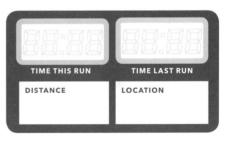

TIME THIS RUN   TIME LAST RUN

DISTANCE   LOCATION

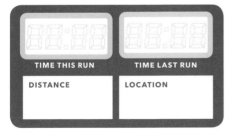

TIME THIS RUN   TIME LAST RUN

DISTANCE   LOCATION

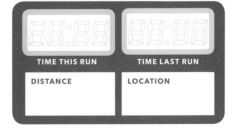

TIME THIS RUN   TIME LAST RUN

DISTANCE   LOCATION

Split Times

Record your split times for races or regular runs.

RACE/RUN NAME					DISTANCE			DATE	
SPLIT NO.	SPLIT NO.	SPLIT NO.	SPLIT NO.	SPLIT NO.	SPLIT NO.	SPLIT NO.	SPLIT NO.	SPLIT NO.	SPLIT NO.
TIME	TIME	TIME	TIME	TIME	TIME	TIME	TIME	TIME	TIME

RACE/RUN NAME					DISTANCE			DATE	
SPLIT NO.	SPLIT NO.	SPLIT NO.	SPLIT NO.	SPLIT NO.	SPLIT NO.	SPLIT NO.	SPLIT NO.	SPLIT NO.	SPLIT NO.
TIME	TIME	TIME	TIME	TIME	TIME	TIME	TIME	TIME	TIME

RACE/RUN NAME					DISTANCE			DATE	
SPLIT NO.	SPLIT NO.	SPLIT NO.	SPLIT NO.	SPLIT NO.	SPLIT NO.	SPLIT NO.	SPLIT NO.	SPLIT NO.	SPLIT NO.
TIME	TIME	TIME	TIME	TIME	TIME	TIME	TIME	TIME	TIME

RACE/RUN NAME					DISTANCE			DATE	
SPLIT NO.	SPLIT NO.	SPLIT NO.	SPLIT NO.	SPLIT NO.	SPLIT NO.	SPLIT NO.	SPLIT NO.	SPLIT NO.	SPLIT NO.
TIME	TIME	TIME	TIME	TIME	TIME	TIME	TIME	TIME	TIME

RACE/RUN NAME					DISTANCE			DATE	
SPLIT NO.	SPLIT NO.	SPLIT NO.	SPLIT NO.	SPLIT NO.	SPLIT NO.	SPLIT NO.	SPLIT NO.	SPLIT NO.	SPLIT NO.
TIME	TIME	TIME	TIME	TIME	TIME	TIME	TIME	TIME	TIME

RACE/RUN NAME					DISTANCE			DATE	
SPLIT NO.	SPLIT NO.	SPLIT NO.	SPLIT NO.	SPLIT NO.	SPLIT NO.	SPLIT NO.	SPLIT NO.	SPLIT NO.	SPLIT NO.
TIME	TIME	TIME	TIME	TIME	TIME	TIME	TIME	TIME	TIME

RACE/RUN NAME					DISTANCE			DATE	
SPLIT NO.	SPLIT NO.	SPLIT NO.	SPLIT NO.	SPLIT NO.	SPLIT NO.	SPLIT NO.	SPLIT NO.	SPLIT NO.	SPLIT NO.
TIME	TIME	TIME	TIME	TIME	TIME	TIME	TIME	TIME	TIME

RACE/RUN NAME					DISTANCE			DATE	
SPLIT NO.	SPLIT NO.	SPLIT NO.	SPLIT NO.	SPLIT NO.	SPLIT NO.	SPLIT NO.	SPLIT NO.	SPLIT NO.	SPLIT NO.
TIME	TIME	TIME	TIME	TIME	TIME	TIME	TIME	TIME	TIME

RACE/RUN NAME					DISTANCE			DATE	
SPLIT NO.	SPLIT NO.	SPLIT NO.	SPLIT NO.	SPLIT NO.	SPLIT NO.	SPLIT NO.	SPLIT NO.	SPLIT NO.	SPLIT NO.
TIME	TIME	TIME	TIME	TIME	TIME	TIME	TIME	TIME	TIME

RACE/RUN NAME					DISTANCE			DATE	
SPLIT NO.	SPLIT NO.	SPLIT NO.	SPLIT NO.	SPLIT NO.	SPLIT NO.	SPLIT NO.	SPLIT NO.	SPLIT NO.	SPLIT NO.
TIME	TIME	TIME	TIME	TIME	TIME	TIME	TIME	TIME	TIME

RACE/RUN NAME					DISTANCE			DATE	
SPLIT NO.	SPLIT NO.	SPLIT NO.	SPLIT NO.	SPLIT NO.	SPLIT NO.	SPLIT NO.	SPLIT NO.	SPLIT NO.	SPLIT NO.
TIME	TIME	TIME	TIME	TIME	TIME	TIME	TIME	TIME	TIME

The Year in Mileage

Color in the miles you run week by week to create
a picture of the total distance you've run this year.

DISTANCE (MILES)

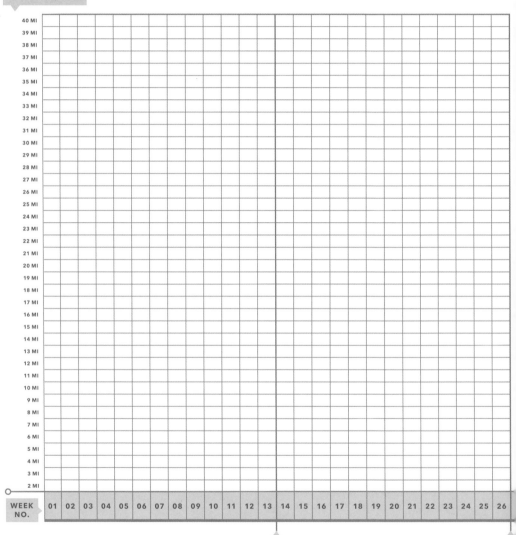

40 MI																									
39 MI																									
38 MI																									
37 MI																									

WEEK NO. 01 02 03 04 05 06 07 08 09 10 11 12 13 14 15 16 17 18 19 20 21 22 23 24 25 26

TOTAL DISTANCE THIS QUARTER

TOTAL DISTANCE THIS QUARTER

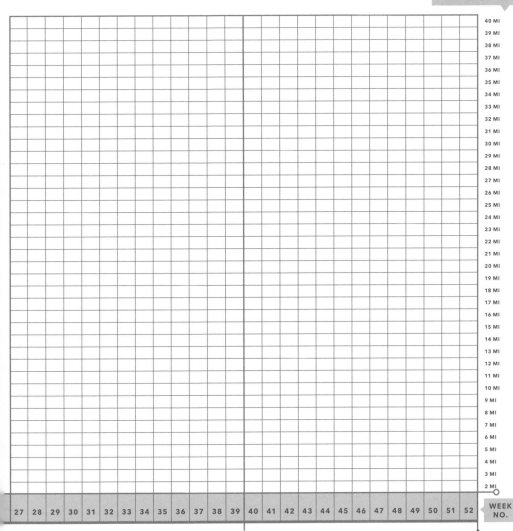

40 MI
39 MI
38 MI
37 MI
36 MI
35 MI
34 MI
33 MI
32 MI
31 MI
30 MI
29 MI
28 MI
27 MI
26 MI
25 MI
24 MI
23 MI
22 MI
21 MI
20 MI
19 MI
18 MI
17 MI
16 MI
15 MI
14 MI
13 MI
12 MI
11 MI
10 MI
9 MI
8 MI
7 MI
6 MI
5 MI
4 MI
3 MI
2 MI

27	28	29	30	31	32	33	34	35	36	37	38	39	40	41	42	43	44	45	46	47	48	49	50	51	52	WEEK NO.

TOTAL DISTANCE
THIS QUARTER

TOTAL DISTANCE
THIS YEAR

The Year in Kilometers

Color in the kilometers you run week by week to create
a picture of the total distance you've run this year.

DISTANCE (KILOMETERS)

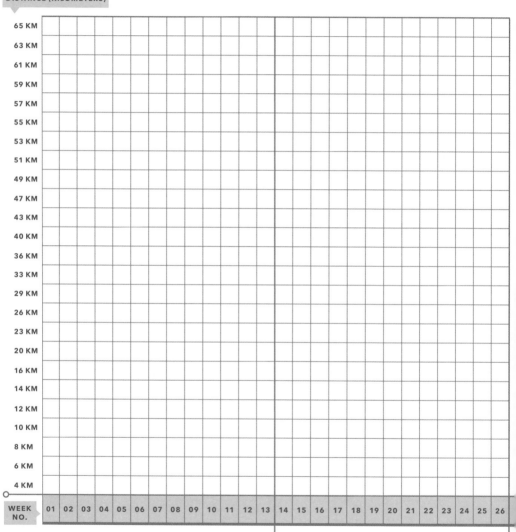

| | TOTAL DISTANCE THIS QUARTER | | TOTAL DISTANCE THIS QUARTER |

	65 KM
	63 KM
	61 KM
	59 KM
	57 KM
	55 KM
	53 KM
	51 KM
	49 KM
	47 KM
	43 KM
	40 KM
	36 KM
	33 KM
	29 KM
	26 KM
	23 KM
	20 KM
	16 KM
	14 KM
	12 KM
	10 KM
	8 KM
	6 KM
	4 KM

27	28	29	30	31	32	33	34	35	36	37	38	39	40	41	42	43	44	45	46	47	48	49	50	51	52	WEEK NO.

TOTAL DISTANCE THIS QUARTER

TOTAL DISTANCE THIS YEAR

WEEK 1

BEGIN DATE

END DATE

TOTAL MILEAGE THIS WEEK

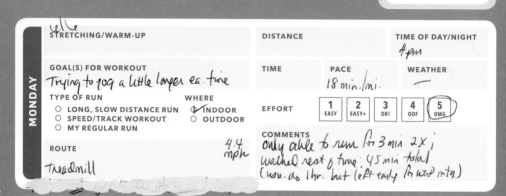

MONDAY

6/6

STRETCHING/WARM-UP

DISTANCE

TIME OF DAY/NIGHT
4pm

GOAL(S) FOR WORKOUT
Trying to jog a little longer ea. time

TIME

PACE
18 min./mi.

WEATHER

TYPE OF RUN
- ○ LONG, SLOW DISTANCE RUN
- ○ SPEED/TRACK WORKOUT
- ○ MY REGULAR RUN

WHERE
- ☑ INDOOR
- ○ OUTDOOR

EFFORT

1 EASY	2 EASY+	3 OK!	4 OOF	5 OMG
				(circled)

ROUTE
Treadmill   *4.4 mph*

COMMENTS
*only able to run for 3 min 2X;
walked rest of time; 45 min total
(usu. do 1 hr. but left early b/c was mtg.)*

TUESDAY

STRETCHING/WARM-UP

DISTANCE

TIME OF DAY/NIGHT

GOAL(S) FOR WORKOUT

TIME

PACE

WEATHER

TYPE OF RUN
- ○ LONG, SLOW DISTANCE RUN
- ○ SPEED/TRACK WORKOUT
- ○ MY REGULAR RUN

WHERE
- ○ INDOOR
- ○ OUTDOOR

EFFORT

1 EASY	2 EASY+	3 OK!	4 OOF	5 OMG

COMMENTS

ROUTE

WEDNESDAY

6/8

STRETCHING/WARM-UP

DISTANCE

TIME OF DAY/NIGHT

GOAL(S) FOR WORKOUT
trying to jog a little longer

TIME

PACE

WEATHER

TYPE OF RUN
- ○ LONG, SLOW DISTANCE RUN
- ○ SPEED/TRACK WORKOUT
- ○ MY REGULAR RUN

WHERE
- ○ INDOOR
- ○ OUTDOOR

EFFORT

1 EASY	2 EASY+	3 OK!	4 OOF	5 OMG
				(circled)

COMMENTS
*ran 6 min; ran 10 min;
ran 6 min   4.4 mph*

ROUTE
treadmill

THURSDAY

STRETCHING/WARM-UP

DISTANCE

TIME OF DAY/NIGHT

GOAL(S) FOR WORKOUT

TIME   **PACE**   **WEATHER**

TYPE OF RUN
- ○ LONG, SLOW DISTANCE RUN
- ○ SPEED/TRACK WORKOUT
- ○ MY REGULAR RUN

WHERE
- ○ INDOOR
- ○ OUTDOOR

EFFORT

1 EASY	2 EASY+	3 OK!	4 OOF	5 OMG

COMMENTS

ROUTE

FRIDAY

STRETCHING/WARM-UP

DISTANCE

TIME OF DAY/NIGHT

GOAL(S) FOR WORKOUT

TIME   **PACE**   **WEATHER**

TYPE OF RUN
- ○ LONG, SLOW DISTANCE RUN
- ○ SPEED/TRACK WORKOUT
- ○ MY REGULAR RUN

WHERE
- ○ INDOOR
- ○ OUTDOOR

EFFORT

1 EASY	2 EASY+	3 OK!	4 OOF	5 OMG

COMMENTS

ROUTE

SATURDAY

STRETCHING/WARM-UP

DISTANCE

TIME OF DAY/NIGHT

GOAL(S) FOR WORKOUT

TIME   **PACE**   **WEATHER**

TYPE OF RUN
- ○ LONG, SLOW DISTANCE RUN
- ○ SPEED/TRACK WORKOUT
- ○ MY REGULAR RUN

WHERE
- ○ INDOOR
- ○ OUTDOOR

EFFORT

1 EASY	2 EASY+	3 OK!	4 OOF	5 OMG

COMMENTS

ROUTE

SUNDAY

STRETCHING/WARM-UP

DISTANCE

TIME OF DAY/NIGHT

GOAL(S) FOR WORKOUT

TIME   **PACE**   **WEATHER**

TYPE OF RUN
- ○ LONG, SLOW DISTANCE RUN
- ○ SPEED/TRACK WORKOUT
- ○ MY REGULAR RUN

WHERE
- ○ INDOOR
- ○ OUTDOOR

EFFORT

1 EASY	2 EASY+	3 OK!	4 OOF	5 OMG

COMMENTS

ROUTE

WEEK 2

BEGIN DATE	END DATE
6/13	6/19

TOTAL MILEAGE THIS WEEK

MONDAY

STRETCHING/WARM-UP	DISTANCE	TIME OF DAY/NIGHT

GOAL(S) FOR WORKOUT	TIME	PACE	WEATHER

TYPE OF RUN
- ○ LONG, SLOW DISTANCE RUN
- ○ SPEED/TRACK WORKOUT
- ○ MY REGULAR RUN

WHERE
- ○ INDOOR
- ○ OUTDOOR

EFFORT: 1 EASY | 2 EASY+ | 3 OK! | 4 OOF | 5 OMG

COMMENTS

ROUTE

TUESDAY

6/14/16

STRETCHING/WARM-UP	DISTANCE	TIME OF DAY/NIGHT

GOAL(S) FOR WORKOUT	TIME	PACE	WEATHER

aerobics – can't job to gym

TYPE OF RUN
- ○ LONG, SLOW DISTANCE RUN
- ○ SPEED/TRACK WORKOUT
- ○ MY REGULAR RUN

WHERE
- ● INDOOR
- ○ OUTDOOR

EFFORT: 1 EASY | 2 EASY+ | 3 OK! | ④ OOF | 5 OMG

COMMENTS
1 hr. 20 min

ROUTE

WEDNESDAY

STRETCHING/WARM-UP	DISTANCE	TIME OF DAY/NIGHT

GOAL(S) FOR WORKOUT	TIME	PACE	WEATHER

TYPE OF RUN
- ○ LONG, SLOW DISTANCE RUN
- ○ SPEED/TRACK WORKOUT
- ○ MY REGULAR RUN

WHERE
- ○ INDOOR
- ○ OUTDOOR

EFFORT: 1 EASY | 2 EASY+ | 3 OK! | 4 OOF | 5 OMG

COMMENTS

ROUTE

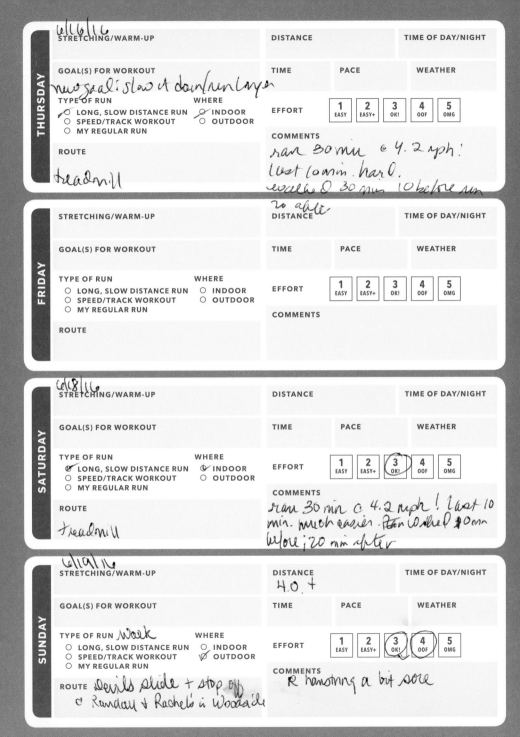

THURSDAY

6/16/16

STRETCHING/WARM-UP

GOAL(S) FOR WORKOUT
new goal: slow it down/run longer

TYPE OF RUN
- ☑ LONG, SLOW DISTANCE RUN
- ○ SPEED/TRACK WORKOUT
- ○ MY REGULAR RUN

WHERE
- ☑ INDOOR
- ○ OUTDOOR

ROUTE
treadmill

DISTANCE

TIME OF DAY/NIGHT

TIME

PACE

WEATHER

EFFORT

| 1 EASY | 2 EASY+ | 3 OK! | 4 OOF | 5 OMG |

COMMENTS
ran 30 min @ 4.2 mph!
last 10 min. hard.
walked @ 30 min 10 before run
20 able

FRIDAY

STRETCHING/WARM-UP

GOAL(S) FOR WORKOUT

TYPE OF RUN
- ○ LONG, SLOW DISTANCE RUN
- ○ SPEED/TRACK WORKOUT
- ○ MY REGULAR RUN

WHERE
- ○ INDOOR
- ○ OUTDOOR

ROUTE

DISTANCE

TIME OF DAY/NIGHT

TIME

PACE

WEATHER

EFFORT

| 1 EASY | 2 EASY+ | 3 OK! | 4 OOF | 5 OMG |

COMMENTS

SATURDAY

6/18/16

STRETCHING/WARM-UP

GOAL(S) FOR WORKOUT

TYPE OF RUN
- ☑ LONG, SLOW DISTANCE RUN
- ○ SPEED/TRACK WORKOUT
- ○ MY REGULAR RUN

WHERE
- ☑ INDOOR
- ○ OUTDOOR

ROUTE
treadmill

DISTANCE

TIME OF DAY/NIGHT

TIME

PACE

WEATHER

EFFORT

| 1 EASY | 2 EASY+ | ③ OK! | 4 OOF | 5 OMG |

COMMENTS
ran 30 min @ 4.2 mph! last 10
min. much easier. Then walked 10 min
before; 20 min after

SUNDAY

6/19/16

STRETCHING/WARM-UP

GOAL(S) FOR WORKOUT

TYPE OF RUN Walk
- ○ LONG, SLOW DISTANCE RUN
- ○ SPEED/TRACK WORKOUT
- ○ MY REGULAR RUN

WHERE
- ○ INDOOR
- ☑ OUTDOOR

ROUTE Devils slide + stop off
@ Randall + Rachel's in Woodside

DISTANCE
4.0 +

TIME OF DAY/NIGHT

TIME

PACE

WEATHER

EFFORT

| 1 EASY | 2 EASY+ | ③ OK! | ④ OOF | 5 OMG |

COMMENTS
R hamstring a bit sore

WEEK 3

BEGIN DATE

END DATE

TOTAL MILEAGE THIS WEEK

MONDAY

STRETCHING/WARM-UP

GOAL(S) FOR WORKOUT

TYPE OF RUN
- ○ LONG, SLOW DISTANCE RUN
- ○ SPEED/TRACK WORKOUT
- ○ MY REGULAR RUN

WHERE
- ○ INDOOR
- ○ OUTDOOR

ROUTE

DISTANCE

TIME OF DAY/NIGHT

TIME

PACE

WEATHER

EFFORT

| 1 EASY | 2 EASY+ | 3 OK! | 4 OOF | 5 OMG |

COMMENTS

TUESDAY

STRETCHING/WARM-UP

GOAL(S) FOR WORKOUT

TYPE OF RUN
- ○ LONG, SLOW DISTANCE RUN
- ○ SPEED/TRACK WORKOUT
- ○ MY REGULAR RUN

WHERE
- ○ INDOOR
- ○ OUTDOOR

ROUTE

DISTANCE

TIME OF DAY/NIGHT

TIME

PACE

WEATHER

EFFORT

| 1 EASY | 2 EASY+ | 3 OK! | 4 OOF | 5 OMG |

COMMENTS

WEDNESDAY

STRETCHING/WARM-UP

GOAL(S) FOR WORKOUT

TYPE OF RUN
- ○ LONG, SLOW DISTANCE RUN
- ○ SPEED/TRACK WORKOUT
- ○ MY REGULAR RUN

WHERE
- ○ INDOOR
- ○ OUTDOOR

ROUTE

DISTANCE

TIME OF DAY/NIGHT

TIME

PACE

WEATHER

EFFORT

| 1 EASY | 2 EASY+ | 3 OK! | 4 OOF | 5 OMG |

COMMENTS

THURSDAY

STRETCHING/WARM-UP

GOAL(S) FOR WORKOUT

TYPE OF RUN
○ LONG, SLOW DISTANCE RUN
○ SPEED/TRACK WORKOUT
○ MY REGULAR RUN

WHERE
○ INDOOR
○ OUTDOOR

ROUTE

DISTANCE

TIME OF DAY/NIGHT

TIME   PACE   WEATHER

EFFORT | 1 EASY | 2 EASY+ | 3 OK! | 4 OOF | 5 OMG |

COMMENTS

FRIDAY

STRETCHING/WARM-UP

GOAL(S) FOR WORKOUT

TYPE OF RUN
○ LONG, SLOW DISTANCE RUN
○ SPEED/TRACK WORKOUT
○ MY REGULAR RUN

WHERE
○ INDOOR
○ OUTDOOR

ROUTE

DISTANCE

TIME OF DAY/NIGHT

TIME   PACE   WEATHER

EFFORT | 1 EASY | 2 EASY+ | 3 OK! | 4 OOF | 5 OMG |

COMMENTS

SATURDAY

STRETCHING/WARM-UP

GOAL(S) FOR WORKOUT

TYPE OF RUN
○ LONG, SLOW DISTANCE RUN
○ SPEED/TRACK WORKOUT
○ MY REGULAR RUN

WHERE
○ INDOOR
○ OUTDOOR

ROUTE

DISTANCE

TIME OF DAY/NIGHT

TIME   PACE   WEATHER

EFFORT | 1 EASY | 2 EASY+ | 3 OK! | 4 OOF | 5 OMG |

COMMENTS

SUNDAY

STRETCHING/WARM-UP

GOAL(S) FOR WORKOUT

TYPE OF RUN
○ LONG, SLOW DISTANCE RUN
○ SPEED/TRACK WORKOUT
○ MY REGULAR RUN

WHERE
○ INDOOR
○ OUTDOOR

ROUTE

DISTANCE

TIME OF DAY/NIGHT

TIME   PACE   WEATHER

EFFORT | 1 EASY | 2 EASY+ | 3 OK! | 4 OOF | 5 OMG |

COMMENTS

WEEK 4

BEGIN DATE

END DATE

TOTAL MILEAGE THIS WEEK

MONDAY

STRETCHING/WARM-UP

GOAL(S) FOR WORKOUT

TYPE OF RUN
- ○ LONG, SLOW DISTANCE RUN
- ○ SPEED/TRACK WORKOUT
- ○ MY REGULAR RUN

WHERE
- ○ INDOOR
- ○ OUTDOOR

ROUTE

DISTANCE

TIME OF DAY/NIGHT

TIME

PACE

WEATHER

EFFORT

| 1 EASY | 2 EASY+ | 3 OK! | 4 OOF | 5 OMG |

COMMENTS

TUESDAY

STRETCHING/WARM-UP

GOAL(S) FOR WORKOUT

TYPE OF RUN
- ○ LONG, SLOW DISTANCE RUN
- ○ SPEED/TRACK WORKOUT
- ○ MY REGULAR RUN

WHERE
- ○ INDOOR
- ○ OUTDOOR

ROUTE

DISTANCE

TIME OF DAY/NIGHT

TIME

PACE

WEATHER

EFFORT

| 1 EASY | 2 EASY+ | 3 OK! | 4 OOF | 5 OMG |

COMMENTS

WEDNESDAY

STRETCHING/WARM-UP

GOAL(S) FOR WORKOUT

TYPE OF RUN
- ○ LONG, SLOW DISTANCE RUN
- ○ SPEED/TRACK WORKOUT
- ○ MY REGULAR RUN

WHERE
- ○ INDOOR
- ○ OUTDOOR

ROUTE

DISTANCE

TIME OF DAY/NIGHT

TIME

PACE

WEATHER

EFFORT

| 1 EASY | 2 EASY+ | 3 OK! | 4 OOF | 5 OMG |

COMMENTS

THURSDAY

STRETCHING/WARM-UP

GOAL(S) FOR WORKOUT

TYPE OF RUN
- ○ LONG, SLOW DISTANCE RUN
- ○ SPEED/TRACK WORKOUT
- ○ MY REGULAR RUN

WHERE
- ○ INDOOR
- ○ OUTDOOR

ROUTE

DISTANCE

TIME OF DAY/NIGHT

TIME

PACE

WEATHER

EFFORT

| 1 EASY | 2 EASY+ | 3 OK! | 4 OOF | 5 OMG |

COMMENTS

FRIDAY

STRETCHING/WARM-UP

GOAL(S) FOR WORKOUT

TYPE OF RUN
- ○ LONG, SLOW DISTANCE RUN
- ○ SPEED/TRACK WORKOUT
- ○ MY REGULAR RUN

WHERE
- ○ INDOOR
- ○ OUTDOOR

ROUTE

DISTANCE

TIME OF DAY/NIGHT

TIME

PACE

WEATHER

EFFORT

| 1 EASY | 2 EASY+ | 3 OK! | 4 OOF | 5 OMG |

COMMENTS

SATURDAY

STRETCHING/WARM-UP

GOAL(S) FOR WORKOUT

TYPE OF RUN
- ○ LONG, SLOW DISTANCE RUN
- ○ SPEED/TRACK WORKOUT
- ○ MY REGULAR RUN

WHERE
- ○ INDOOR
- ○ OUTDOOR

ROUTE

DISTANCE

TIME OF DAY/NIGHT

TIME

PACE

WEATHER

EFFORT

| 1 EASY | 2 EASY+ | 3 OK! | 4 OOF | 5 OMG |

COMMENTS

SUNDAY

STRETCHING/WARM-UP

GOAL(S) FOR WORKOUT

TYPE OF RUN
- ○ LONG, SLOW DISTANCE RUN
- ○ SPEED/TRACK WORKOUT
- ○ MY REGULAR RUN

WHERE
- ○ INDOOR
- ○ OUTDOOR

ROUTE

DISTANCE

TIME OF DAY/NIGHT

TIME

PACE

WEATHER

EFFORT

| 1 EASY | 2 EASY+ | 3 OK! | 4 OOF | 5 OMG |

COMMENTS

WEEK 5

BEGIN DATE

END DATE

TOTAL MILEAGE THIS WEEK

MONDAY

STRETCHING/WARM-UP

GOAL(S) FOR WORKOUT

TYPE OF RUN
- ○ LONG, SLOW DISTANCE RUN
- ○ SPEED/TRACK WORKOUT
- ○ MY REGULAR RUN

WHERE
- ○ INDOOR
- ○ OUTDOOR

ROUTE

DISTANCE

TIME OF DAY/NIGHT

TIME

PACE

WEATHER

EFFORT

| 1 EASY | 2 EASY+ | 3 OK! | 4 OOF | 5 OMG |

COMMENTS

TUESDAY

STRETCHING/WARM-UP

GOAL(S) FOR WORKOUT

TYPE OF RUN
- ○ LONG, SLOW DISTANCE RUN
- ○ SPEED/TRACK WORKOUT
- ○ MY REGULAR RUN

WHERE
- ○ INDOOR
- ○ OUTDOOR

ROUTE

DISTANCE

TIME OF DAY/NIGHT

TIME

PACE

WEATHER

EFFORT

| 1 EASY | 2 EASY+ | 3 OK! | 4 OOF | 5 OMG |

COMMENTS

WEDNESDAY

STRETCHING/WARM-UP

GOAL(S) FOR WORKOUT

TYPE OF RUN
- ○ LONG, SLOW DISTANCE RUN
- ○ SPEED/TRACK WORKOUT
- ○ MY REGULAR RUN

WHERE
- ○ INDOOR
- ○ OUTDOOR

ROUTE

DISTANCE

TIME OF DAY/NIGHT

TIME

PACE

WEATHER

EFFORT

| 1 EASY | 2 EASY+ | 3 OK! | 4 OOF | 5 OMG |

COMMENTS

THURSDAY

STRETCHING/WARM-UP

GOAL(S) FOR WORKOUT

TYPE OF RUN
- ○ LONG, SLOW DISTANCE RUN
- ○ SPEED/TRACK WORKOUT
- ○ MY REGULAR RUN

WHERE
- ○ INDOOR
- ○ OUTDOOR

ROUTE

DISTANCE

TIME OF DAY/NIGHT

TIME

PACE

WEATHER

EFFORT

1	2	3	4	5
EASY	EASY+	OK!	OOF	OMG

COMMENTS

FRIDAY

STRETCHING/WARM-UP

GOAL(S) FOR WORKOUT

TYPE OF RUN
- ○ LONG, SLOW DISTANCE RUN
- ○ SPEED/TRACK WORKOUT
- ○ MY REGULAR RUN

WHERE
- ○ INDOOR
- ○ OUTDOOR

ROUTE

DISTANCE

TIME OF DAY/NIGHT

TIME

PACE

WEATHER

EFFORT

1	2	3	4	5
EASY	EASY+	OK!	OOF	OMG

COMMENTS

SATURDAY

STRETCHING/WARM-UP

GOAL(S) FOR WORKOUT

TYPE OF RUN
- ○ LONG, SLOW DISTANCE RUN
- ○ SPEED/TRACK WORKOUT
- ○ MY REGULAR RUN

WHERE
- ○ INDOOR
- ○ OUTDOOR

ROUTE

DISTANCE

TIME OF DAY/NIGHT

TIME

PACE

WEATHER

EFFORT

1	2	3	4	5
EASY	EASY+	OK!	OOF	OMG

COMMENTS

SUNDAY

STRETCHING/WARM-UP

GOAL(S) FOR WORKOUT

TYPE OF RUN
- ○ LONG, SLOW DISTANCE RUN
- ○ SPEED/TRACK WORKOUT
- ○ MY REGULAR RUN

WHERE
- ○ INDOOR
- ○ OUTDOOR

ROUTE

DISTANCE

TIME OF DAY/NIGHT

TIME

PACE

WEATHER

EFFORT

1	2	3	4	5
EASY	EASY+	OK!	OOF	OMG

COMMENTS

WEEK 6

BEGIN DATE

END DATE

TOTAL MILEAGE THIS WEEK

MONDAY

STRETCHING/WARM-UP

GOAL(S) FOR WORKOUT

TYPE OF RUN
- ○ LONG, SLOW DISTANCE RUN
- ○ SPEED/TRACK WORKOUT
- ○ MY REGULAR RUN

WHERE
- ○ INDOOR
- ○ OUTDOOR

ROUTE

DISTANCE

TIME OF DAY/NIGHT

TIME   PACE   WEATHER

EFFORT
| 1 EASY | 2 EASY+ | 3 OK! | 4 OOF | 5 OMG |

COMMENTS

TUESDAY

STRETCHING/WARM-UP

GOAL(S) FOR WORKOUT

TYPE OF RUN
- ○ LONG, SLOW DISTANCE RUN
- ○ SPEED/TRACK WORKOUT
- ○ MY REGULAR RUN

WHERE
- ○ INDOOR
- ○ OUTDOOR

ROUTE

DISTANCE

TIME OF DAY/NIGHT

TIME   PACE   WEATHER

EFFORT
| 1 EASY | 2 EASY+ | 3 OK! | 4 OOF | 5 OMG |

COMMENTS

WEDNESDAY

STRETCHING/WARM-UP

GOAL(S) FOR WORKOUT

TYPE OF RUN
- ○ LONG, SLOW DISTANCE RUN
- ○ SPEED/TRACK WORKOUT
- ○ MY REGULAR RUN

WHERE
- ○ INDOOR
- ○ OUTDOOR

ROUTE

DISTANCE

TIME OF DAY/NIGHT

TIME   PACE   WEATHER

EFFORT
| 1 EASY | 2 EASY+ | 3 OK! | 4 OOF | 5 OMG |

COMMENTS

THURSDAY

STRETCHING/WARM-UP

DISTANCE

TIME OF DAY/NIGHT

GOAL(S) FOR WORKOUT

TIME　　**PACE**　　**WEATHER**

TYPE OF RUN
- ○ LONG, SLOW DISTANCE RUN
- ○ SPEED/TRACK WORKOUT
- ○ MY REGULAR RUN

WHERE
- ○ INDOOR
- ○ OUTDOOR

EFFORT

1 EASY	2 EASY+	3 OK!	4 OOF	5 OMG

COMMENTS

ROUTE

FRIDAY

STRETCHING/WARM-UP

DISTANCE

TIME OF DAY/NIGHT

GOAL(S) FOR WORKOUT

TIME　　**PACE**　　**WEATHER**

TYPE OF RUN
- ○ LONG, SLOW DISTANCE RUN
- ○ SPEED/TRACK WORKOUT
- ○ MY REGULAR RUN

WHERE
- ○ INDOOR
- ○ OUTDOOR

EFFORT

1 EASY	2 EASY+	3 OK!	4 OOF	5 OMG

COMMENTS

ROUTE

SATURDAY

STRETCHING/WARM-UP

DISTANCE

TIME OF DAY/NIGHT

GOAL(S) FOR WORKOUT

TIME　　**PACE**　　**WEATHER**

TYPE OF RUN
- ○ LONG, SLOW DISTANCE RUN
- ○ SPEED/TRACK WORKOUT
- ○ MY REGULAR RUN

WHERE
- ○ INDOOR
- ○ OUTDOOR

EFFORT

1 EASY	2 EASY+	3 OK!	4 OOF	5 OMG

COMMENTS

ROUTE

SUNDAY

STRETCHING/WARM-UP

DISTANCE

TIME OF DAY/NIGHT

GOAL(S) FOR WORKOUT

TIME　　**PACE**　　**WEATHER**

TYPE OF RUN
- ○ LONG, SLOW DISTANCE RUN
- ○ SPEED/TRACK WORKOUT
- ○ MY REGULAR RUN

WHERE
- ○ INDOOR
- ○ OUTDOOR

EFFORT

1 EASY	2 EASY+	3 OK!	4 OOF	5 OMG

COMMENTS

ROUTE

WEEK 7

BEGIN DATE

END DATE

TOTAL MILEAGE THIS WEEK

MONDAY

STRETCHING/WARM-UP

DISTANCE

TIME OF DAY/NIGHT

GOAL(S) FOR WORKOUT

TIME

PACE

WEATHER

TYPE OF RUN
- LONG, SLOW DISTANCE RUN
- SPEED/TRACK WORKOUT
- MY REGULAR RUN

WHERE
- INDOOR
- OUTDOOR

EFFORT

| 1 EASY | 2 EASY+ | 3 OK! | 4 OOF | 5 OMG |

COMMENTS

ROUTE

TUESDAY

STRETCHING/WARM-UP

DISTANCE

TIME OF DAY/NIGHT

GOAL(S) FOR WORKOUT

TIME

PACE

WEATHER

TYPE OF RUN
- LONG, SLOW DISTANCE RUN
- SPEED/TRACK WORKOUT
- MY REGULAR RUN

WHERE
- INDOOR
- OUTDOOR

EFFORT

| 1 EASY | 2 EASY+ | 3 OK! | 4 OOF | 5 OMG |

COMMENTS

ROUTE

WEDNESDAY

STRETCHING/WARM-UP

DISTANCE

TIME OF DAY/NIGHT

GOAL(S) FOR WORKOUT

TIME

PACE

WEATHER

TYPE OF RUN
- LONG, SLOW DISTANCE RUN
- SPEED/TRACK WORKOUT
- MY REGULAR RUN

WHERE
- INDOOR
- OUTDOOR

EFFORT

| 1 EASY | 2 EASY+ | 3 OK! | 4 OOF | 5 OMG |

COMMENTS

ROUTE

THURSDAY

STRETCHING/WARM-UP

GOAL(S) FOR WORKOUT

TYPE OF RUN
- ○ LONG, SLOW DISTANCE RUN
- ○ SPEED/TRACK WORKOUT
- ○ MY REGULAR RUN

WHERE
- ○ INDOOR
- ○ OUTDOOR

ROUTE

DISTANCE

TIME OF DAY/NIGHT

TIME

PACE

WEATHER

EFFORT

1 EASY	2 EASY+	3 OK!	4 OOF	5 OMG

COMMENTS

FRIDAY

STRETCHING/WARM-UP

GOAL(S) FOR WORKOUT

TYPE OF RUN
- ○ LONG, SLOW DISTANCE RUN
- ○ SPEED/TRACK WORKOUT
- ○ MY REGULAR RUN

WHERE
- ○ INDOOR
- ○ OUTDOOR

ROUTE

DISTANCE

TIME OF DAY/NIGHT

TIME

PACE

WEATHER

EFFORT

1 EASY	2 EASY+	3 OK!	4 OOF	5 OMG

COMMENTS

SATURDAY

STRETCHING/WARM-UP

GOAL(S) FOR WORKOUT

TYPE OF RUN
- ○ LONG, SLOW DISTANCE RUN
- ○ SPEED/TRACK WORKOUT
- ○ MY REGULAR RUN

WHERE
- ○ INDOOR
- ○ OUTDOOR

ROUTE

DISTANCE

TIME OF DAY/NIGHT

TIME

PACE

WEATHER

EFFORT

1 EASY	2 EASY+	3 OK!	4 OOF	5 OMG

COMMENTS

SUNDAY

STRETCHING/WARM-UP

GOAL(S) FOR WORKOUT

TYPE OF RUN
- ○ LONG, SLOW DISTANCE RUN
- ○ SPEED/TRACK WORKOUT
- ○ MY REGULAR RUN

WHERE
- ○ INDOOR
- ○ OUTDOOR

ROUTE

DISTANCE

TIME OF DAY/NIGHT

TIME

PACE

WEATHER

EFFORT

1 EASY	2 EASY+	3 OK!	4 OOF	5 OMG

COMMENTS

WEEK 8

BEGIN DATE	END DATE

TOTAL MILEAGE THIS WEEK

MONDAY

STRETCHING/WARM-UP

GOAL(S) FOR WORKOUT

TYPE OF RUN
- ○ LONG, SLOW DISTANCE RUN
- ○ SPEED/TRACK WORKOUT
- ○ MY REGULAR RUN

WHERE
- ○ INDOOR
- ○ OUTDOOR

ROUTE

DISTANCE

TIME OF DAY/NIGHT

TIME

PACE

WEATHER

EFFORT

1 EASY	2 EASY+	3 OK!	4 OOF	5 OMG

COMMENTS

TUESDAY

STRETCHING/WARM-UP

GOAL(S) FOR WORKOUT

TYPE OF RUN
- ○ LONG, SLOW DISTANCE RUN
- ○ SPEED/TRACK WORKOUT
- ○ MY REGULAR RUN

WHERE
- ○ INDOOR
- ○ OUTDOOR

ROUTE

DISTANCE

TIME OF DAY/NIGHT

TIME

PACE

WEATHER

EFFORT

1 EASY	2 EASY+	3 OK!	4 OOF	5 OMG

COMMENTS

WEDNESDAY

STRETCHING/WARM-UP

GOAL(S) FOR WORKOUT

TYPE OF RUN
- ○ LONG, SLOW DISTANCE RUN
- ○ SPEED/TRACK WORKOUT
- ○ MY REGULAR RUN

WHERE
- ○ INDOOR
- ○ OUTDOOR

ROUTE

DISTANCE

TIME OF DAY/NIGHT

TIME

PACE

WEATHER

EFFORT

1 EASY	2 EASY+	3 OK!	4 OOF	5 OMG

COMMENTS

THURSDAY

STRETCHING/WARM-UP

GOAL(S) FOR WORKOUT

TYPE OF RUN
- ○ LONG, SLOW DISTANCE RUN
- ○ SPEED/TRACK WORKOUT
- ○ MY REGULAR RUN

WHERE
- ○ INDOOR
- ○ OUTDOOR

ROUTE

DISTANCE

TIME OF DAY/NIGHT

TIME

PACE

WEATHER

EFFORT

1 EASY	2 EASY+	3 OK!	4 OOF	5 OMG

COMMENTS

FRIDAY

STRETCHING/WARM-UP

GOAL(S) FOR WORKOUT

TYPE OF RUN
- ○ LONG, SLOW DISTANCE RUN
- ○ SPEED/TRACK WORKOUT
- ○ MY REGULAR RUN

WHERE
- ○ INDOOR
- ○ OUTDOOR

ROUTE

DISTANCE

TIME OF DAY/NIGHT

TIME

PACE

WEATHER

EFFORT

1 EASY	2 EASY+	3 OK!	4 OOF	5 OMG

COMMENTS

SATURDAY

STRETCHING/WARM-UP

GOAL(S) FOR WORKOUT

TYPE OF RUN
- ○ LONG, SLOW DISTANCE RUN
- ○ SPEED/TRACK WORKOUT
- ○ MY REGULAR RUN

WHERE
- ○ INDOOR
- ○ OUTDOOR

ROUTE

DISTANCE

TIME OF DAY/NIGHT

TIME

PACE

WEATHER

EFFORT

1 EASY	2 EASY+	3 OK!	4 OOF	5 OMG

COMMENTS

SUNDAY

STRETCHING/WARM-UP

GOAL(S) FOR WORKOUT

TYPE OF RUN
- ○ LONG, SLOW DISTANCE RUN
- ○ SPEED/TRACK WORKOUT
- ○ MY REGULAR RUN

WHERE
- ○ INDOOR
- ○ OUTDOOR

ROUTE

DISTANCE

TIME OF DAY/NIGHT

TIME

PACE

WEATHER

EFFORT

1 EASY	2 EASY+	3 OK!	4 OOF	5 OMG

COMMENTS

WEEK 9

BEGIN DATE

END DATE

TOTAL MILEAGE THIS WEEK

MONDAY

STRETCHING/WARM-UP

GOAL(S) FOR WORKOUT

TYPE OF RUN
- ○ LONG, SLOW DISTANCE RUN
- ○ SPEED/TRACK WORKOUT
- ○ MY REGULAR RUN

WHERE
- ○ INDOOR
- ○ OUTDOOR

ROUTE

DISTANCE

TIME OF DAY/NIGHT

TIME

PACE

WEATHER

EFFORT

| 1 EASY | 2 EASY+ | 3 OK! | 4 OOF | 5 OMG |

COMMENTS

TUESDAY

STRETCHING/WARM-UP

GOAL(S) FOR WORKOUT

TYPE OF RUN
- ○ LONG, SLOW DISTANCE RUN
- ○ SPEED/TRACK WORKOUT
- ○ MY REGULAR RUN

WHERE
- ○ INDOOR
- ○ OUTDOOR

ROUTE

DISTANCE

TIME OF DAY/NIGHT

TIME

PACE

WEATHER

EFFORT

| 1 EASY | 2 EASY+ | 3 OK! | 4 OOF | 5 OMG |

COMMENTS

WEDNESDAY

STRETCHING/WARM-UP

GOAL(S) FOR WORKOUT

TYPE OF RUN
- ○ LONG, SLOW DISTANCE RUN
- ○ SPEED/TRACK WORKOUT
- ○ MY REGULAR RUN

WHERE
- ○ INDOOR
- ○ OUTDOOR

ROUTE

DISTANCE

TIME OF DAY/NIGHT

TIME

PACE

WEATHER

EFFORT

| 1 EASY | 2 EASY+ | 3 OK! | 4 OOF | 5 OMG |

COMMENTS

THURSDAY

STRETCHING/WARM-UP

DISTANCE

TIME OF DAY/NIGHT

GOAL(S) FOR WORKOUT

TIME

PACE

WEATHER

TYPE OF RUN
- ○ LONG, SLOW DISTANCE RUN
- ○ SPEED/TRACK WORKOUT
- ○ MY REGULAR RUN

WHERE
- ○ INDOOR
- ○ OUTDOOR

EFFORT

| 1 EASY | 2 EASY+ | 3 OK! | 4 OOF | 5 OMG |

COMMENTS

ROUTE

FRIDAY

STRETCHING/WARM-UP

DISTANCE

TIME OF DAY/NIGHT

GOAL(S) FOR WORKOUT

TIME

PACE

WEATHER

TYPE OF RUN
- ○ LONG, SLOW DISTANCE RUN
- ○ SPEED/TRACK WORKOUT
- ○ MY REGULAR RUN

WHERE
- ○ INDOOR
- ○ OUTDOOR

EFFORT

| 1 EASY | 2 EASY+ | 3 OK! | 4 OOF | 5 OMG |

COMMENTS

ROUTE

SATURDAY

STRETCHING/WARM-UP

DISTANCE

TIME OF DAY/NIGHT

GOAL(S) FOR WORKOUT

TIME

PACE

WEATHER

TYPE OF RUN
- ○ LONG, SLOW DISTANCE RUN
- ○ SPEED/TRACK WORKOUT
- ○ MY REGULAR RUN

WHERE
- ○ INDOOR
- ○ OUTDOOR

EFFORT

| 1 EASY | 2 EASY+ | 3 OK! | 4 OOF | 5 OMG |

COMMENTS

ROUTE

SUNDAY

STRETCHING/WARM-UP

DISTANCE

TIME OF DAY/NIGHT

GOAL(S) FOR WORKOUT

TIME

PACE

WEATHER

TYPE OF RUN
- ○ LONG, SLOW DISTANCE RUN
- ○ SPEED/TRACK WORKOUT
- ○ MY REGULAR RUN

WHERE
- ○ INDOOR
- ○ OUTDOOR

EFFORT

| 1 EASY | 2 EASY+ | 3 OK! | 4 OOF | 5 OMG |

COMMENTS

ROUTE

WEEK 10

BEGIN DATE

END DATE

TOTAL MILEAGE THIS WEEK

MONDAY

STRETCHING/WARM-UP

DISTANCE

TIME OF DAY/NIGHT

GOAL(S) FOR WORKOUT

TIME

PACE

WEATHER

TYPE OF RUN
- ○ LONG, SLOW DISTANCE RUN
- ○ SPEED/TRACK WORKOUT
- ○ MY REGULAR RUN

WHERE
- ○ INDOOR
- ○ OUTDOOR

EFFORT

| 1 EASY | 2 EASY+ | 3 OK! | 4 OOF | 5 OMG |

COMMENTS

ROUTE

TUESDAY

STRETCHING/WARM-UP

DISTANCE

TIME OF DAY/NIGHT

GOAL(S) FOR WORKOUT

TIME

PACE

WEATHER

TYPE OF RUN
- ○ LONG, SLOW DISTANCE RUN
- ○ SPEED/TRACK WORKOUT
- ○ MY REGULAR RUN

WHERE
- ○ INDOOR
- ○ OUTDOOR

EFFORT

| 1 EASY | 2 EASY+ | 3 OK! | 4 OOF | 5 OMG |

COMMENTS

ROUTE

WEDNESDAY

STRETCHING/WARM-UP

DISTANCE

TIME OF DAY/NIGHT

GOAL(S) FOR WORKOUT

TIME

PACE

WEATHER

TYPE OF RUN
- ○ LONG, SLOW DISTANCE RUN
- ○ SPEED/TRACK WORKOUT
- ○ MY REGULAR RUN

WHERE
- ○ INDOOR
- ○ OUTDOOR

EFFORT

| 1 EASY | 2 EASY+ | 3 OK! | 4 OOF | 5 OMG |

COMMENTS

ROUTE

THURSDAY

STRETCHING/WARM-UP

GOAL(S) FOR WORKOUT

TYPE OF RUN
○ LONG, SLOW DISTANCE RUN
○ SPEED/TRACK WORKOUT
○ MY REGULAR RUN

WHERE
○ INDOOR
○ OUTDOOR

ROUTE

DISTANCE

TIME OF DAY/NIGHT

TIME

PACE

WEATHER

EFFORT

| 1 EASY | 2 EASY+ | 3 OK! | 4 OOF | 5 OMG |

COMMENTS

FRIDAY

STRETCHING/WARM-UP

GOAL(S) FOR WORKOUT

TYPE OF RUN
○ LONG, SLOW DISTANCE RUN
○ SPEED/TRACK WORKOUT
○ MY REGULAR RUN

WHERE
○ INDOOR
○ OUTDOOR

ROUTE

DISTANCE

TIME OF DAY/NIGHT

TIME

PACE

WEATHER

EFFORT

| 1 EASY | 2 EASY+ | 3 OK! | 4 OOF | 5 OMG |

COMMENTS

SATURDAY

STRETCHING/WARM-UP

GOAL(S) FOR WORKOUT

TYPE OF RUN
○ LONG, SLOW DISTANCE RUN
○ SPEED/TRACK WORKOUT
○ MY REGULAR RUN

WHERE
○ INDOOR
○ OUTDOOR

ROUTE

DISTANCE

TIME OF DAY/NIGHT

TIME

PACE

WEATHER

EFFORT

| 1 EASY | 2 EASY+ | 3 OK! | 4 OOF | 5 OMG |

COMMENTS

SUNDAY

STRETCHING/WARM-UP

GOAL(S) FOR WORKOUT

TYPE OF RUN
○ LONG, SLOW DISTANCE RUN
○ SPEED/TRACK WORKOUT
○ MY REGULAR RUN

WHERE
○ INDOOR
○ OUTDOOR

ROUTE

DISTANCE

TIME OF DAY/NIGHT

TIME

PACE

WEATHER

EFFORT

| 1 EASY | 2 EASY+ | 3 OK! | 4 OOF | 5 OMG |

COMMENTS

WEEK 11

BEGIN DATE

END DATE

TOTAL MILEAGE THIS WEEK

MONDAY

STRETCHING/WARM-UP

GOAL(S) FOR WORKOUT

TYPE OF RUN
- ○ LONG, SLOW DISTANCE RUN
- ○ SPEED/TRACK WORKOUT
- ○ MY REGULAR RUN

WHERE
- ○ INDOOR
- ○ OUTDOOR

ROUTE

DISTANCE

TIME OF DAY/NIGHT

TIME   PACE   WEATHER

EFFORT

| 1 EASY | 2 EASY+ | 3 OK! | 4 OOF | 5 OMG |

COMMENTS

TUESDAY

STRETCHING/WARM-UP

GOAL(S) FOR WORKOUT

TYPE OF RUN
- ○ LONG, SLOW DISTANCE RUN
- ○ SPEED/TRACK WORKOUT
- ○ MY REGULAR RUN

WHERE
- ○ INDOOR
- ○ OUTDOOR

ROUTE

DISTANCE

TIME OF DAY/NIGHT

TIME   PACE   WEATHER

EFFORT

| 1 EASY | 2 EASY+ | 3 OK! | 4 OOF | 5 OMG |

COMMENTS

WEDNESDAY

STRETCHING/WARM-UP

GOAL(S) FOR WORKOUT

TYPE OF RUN
- ○ LONG, SLOW DISTANCE RUN
- ○ SPEED/TRACK WORKOUT
- ○ MY REGULAR RUN

WHERE
- ○ INDOOR
- ○ OUTDOOR

ROUTE

DISTANCE

TIME OF DAY/NIGHT

TIME   PACE   WEATHER

EFFORT

| 1 EASY | 2 EASY+ | 3 OK! | 4 OOF | 5 OMG |

COMMENTS

THURSDAY

STRETCHING/WARM-UP

GOAL(S) FOR WORKOUT

TYPE OF RUN
- ○ LONG, SLOW DISTANCE RUN
- ○ SPEED/TRACK WORKOUT
- ○ MY REGULAR RUN

WHERE
- ○ INDOOR
- ○ OUTDOOR

ROUTE

DISTANCE

TIME OF DAY/NIGHT

TIME

PACE

WEATHER

EFFORT

1 EASY	2 EASY+	3 OK!	4 OOF	5 OMG

COMMENTS

FRIDAY

STRETCHING/WARM-UP

GOAL(S) FOR WORKOUT

TYPE OF RUN
- ○ LONG, SLOW DISTANCE RUN
- ○ SPEED/TRACK WORKOUT
- ○ MY REGULAR RUN

WHERE
- ○ INDOOR
- ○ OUTDOOR

ROUTE

DISTANCE

TIME OF DAY/NIGHT

TIME

PACE

WEATHER

EFFORT

1 EASY	2 EASY+	3 OK!	4 OOF	5 OMG

COMMENTS

SATURDAY

STRETCHING/WARM-UP

GOAL(S) FOR WORKOUT

TYPE OF RUN
- ○ LONG, SLOW DISTANCE RUN
- ○ SPEED/TRACK WORKOUT
- ○ MY REGULAR RUN

WHERE
- ○ INDOOR
- ○ OUTDOOR

ROUTE

DISTANCE

TIME OF DAY/NIGHT

TIME

PACE

WEATHER

EFFORT

1 EASY	2 EASY+	3 OK!	4 OOF	5 OMG

COMMENTS

SUNDAY

STRETCHING/WARM-UP

GOAL(S) FOR WORKOUT

TYPE OF RUN
- ○ LONG, SLOW DISTANCE RUN
- ○ SPEED/TRACK WORKOUT
- ○ MY REGULAR RUN

WHERE
- ○ INDOOR
- ○ OUTDOOR

ROUTE

DISTANCE

TIME OF DAY/NIGHT

TIME

PACE

WEATHER

EFFORT

1 EASY	2 EASY+	3 OK!	4 OOF	5 OMG

COMMENTS

MONDAY

STRETCHING/WARM-UP

DISTANCE

TIME OF DAY/NIGHT

GOAL(S) FOR WORKOUT

TIME

PACE

WEATHER

TYPE OF RUN
- ○ LONG, SLOW DISTANCE RUN
- ○ SPEED/TRACK WORKOUT
- ○ MY REGULAR RUN

WHERE
- ○ INDOOR
- ○ OUTDOOR

EFFORT

| 1 EASY | 2 EASY+ | 3 OK! | 4 OOF | 5 OMG |

COMMENTS

ROUTE

TUESDAY

STRETCHING/WARM-UP

DISTANCE

TIME OF DAY/NIGHT

GOAL(S) FOR WORKOUT

TIME

PACE

WEATHER

TYPE OF RUN
- ○ LONG, SLOW DISTANCE RUN
- ○ SPEED/TRACK WORKOUT
- ○ MY REGULAR RUN

WHERE
- ○ INDOOR
- ○ OUTDOOR

EFFORT

| 1 EASY | 2 EASY+ | 3 OK! | 4 OOF | 5 OMG |

COMMENTS

ROUTE

WEDNESDAY

STRETCHING/WARM-UP

DISTANCE

TIME OF DAY/NIGHT

GOAL(S) FOR WORKOUT

TIME

PACE

WEATHER

TYPE OF RUN
- ○ LONG, SLOW DISTANCE RUN
- ○ SPEED/TRACK WORKOUT
- ○ MY REGULAR RUN

WHERE
- ○ INDOOR
- ○ OUTDOOR

EFFORT

| 1 EASY | 2 EASY+ | 3 OK! | 4 OOF | 5 OMG |

COMMENTS

ROUTE

THURSDAY

STRETCHING/WARM-UP

DISTANCE

TIME OF DAY/NIGHT

GOAL(S) FOR WORKOUT

TIME **PACE** **WEATHER**

TYPE OF RUN
○ LONG, SLOW DISTANCE RUN
○ SPEED/TRACK WORKOUT
○ MY REGULAR RUN

WHERE
○ INDOOR
○ OUTDOOR

EFFORT

| 1 EASY | 2 EASY+ | 3 OK! | 4 OOF | 5 OMG |

COMMENTS

ROUTE

FRIDAY

STRETCHING/WARM-UP

DISTANCE

TIME OF DAY/NIGHT

GOAL(S) FOR WORKOUT

TIME **PACE** **WEATHER**

TYPE OF RUN
○ LONG, SLOW DISTANCE RUN
○ SPEED/TRACK WORKOUT
○ MY REGULAR RUN

WHERE
○ INDOOR
○ OUTDOOR

EFFORT

| 1 EASY | 2 EASY+ | 3 OK! | 4 OOF | 5 OMG |

COMMENTS

ROUTE

SATURDAY

STRETCHING/WARM-UP

DISTANCE

TIME OF DAY/NIGHT

GOAL(S) FOR WORKOUT

TIME **PACE** **WEATHER**

TYPE OF RUN
○ LONG, SLOW DISTANCE RUN
○ SPEED/TRACK WORKOUT
○ MY REGULAR RUN

WHERE
○ INDOOR
○ OUTDOOR

EFFORT

| 1 EASY | 2 EASY+ | 3 OK! | 4 OOF | 5 OMG |

COMMENTS

ROUTE

SUNDAY

STRETCHING/WARM-UP

DISTANCE

TIME OF DAY/NIGHT

GOAL(S) FOR WORKOUT

TIME **PACE** **WEATHER**

TYPE OF RUN
○ LONG, SLOW DISTANCE RUN
○ SPEED/TRACK WORKOUT
○ MY REGULAR RUN

WHERE
○ INDOOR
○ OUTDOOR

EFFORT

| 1 EASY | 2 EASY+ | 3 OK! | 4 OOF | 5 OMG |

COMMENTS

ROUTE

WEEK 13

BEGIN DATE

END DATE

TOTAL MILEAGE THIS WEEK

MONDAY

STRETCHING/WARM-UP

DISTANCE

TIME OF DAY/NIGHT

GOAL(S) FOR WORKOUT

TIME

PACE

WEATHER

TYPE OF RUN
- ○ LONG, SLOW DISTANCE RUN
- ○ SPEED/TRACK WORKOUT
- ○ MY REGULAR RUN

WHERE
- ○ INDOOR
- ○ OUTDOOR

EFFORT

| 1 EASY | 2 EASY+ | 3 OK! | 4 OOF | 5 OMG |

COMMENTS

ROUTE

TUESDAY

STRETCHING/WARM-UP

DISTANCE

TIME OF DAY/NIGHT

GOAL(S) FOR WORKOUT

TIME

PACE

WEATHER

TYPE OF RUN
- ○ LONG, SLOW DISTANCE RUN
- ○ SPEED/TRACK WORKOUT
- ○ MY REGULAR RUN

WHERE
- ○ INDOOR
- ○ OUTDOOR

EFFORT

| 1 EASY | 2 EASY+ | 3 OK! | 4 OOF | 5 OMG |

COMMENTS

ROUTE

WEDNESDAY

STRETCHING/WARM-UP

DISTANCE

TIME OF DAY/NIGHT

GOAL(S) FOR WORKOUT

TIME

PACE

WEATHER

TYPE OF RUN
- ○ LONG, SLOW DISTANCE RUN
- ○ SPEED/TRACK WORKOUT
- ○ MY REGULAR RUN

WHERE
- ○ INDOOR
- ○ OUTDOOR

EFFORT

| 1 EASY | 2 EASY+ | 3 OK! | 4 OOF | 5 OMG |

COMMENTS

ROUTE

THURSDAY

STRETCHING/WARM-UP

GOAL(S) FOR WORKOUT

TYPE OF RUN
- ○ LONG, SLOW DISTANCE RUN
- ○ SPEED/TRACK WORKOUT
- ○ MY REGULAR RUN

WHERE
- ○ INDOOR
- ○ OUTDOOR

ROUTE

DISTANCE

TIME OF DAY/NIGHT

TIME

PACE

WEATHER

EFFORT
| 1 EASY | 2 EASY+ | 3 OK! | 4 OOF | 5 OMG |

COMMENTS

FRIDAY

STRETCHING/WARM-UP

GOAL(S) FOR WORKOUT

TYPE OF RUN
- ○ LONG, SLOW DISTANCE RUN
- ○ SPEED/TRACK WORKOUT
- ○ MY REGULAR RUN

WHERE
- ○ INDOOR
- ○ OUTDOOR

ROUTE

DISTANCE

TIME OF DAY/NIGHT

TIME

PACE

WEATHER

EFFORT
| 1 EASY | 2 EASY+ | 3 OK! | 4 OOF | 5 OMG |

COMMENTS

SATURDAY

STRETCHING/WARM-UP

GOAL(S) FOR WORKOUT

TYPE OF RUN
- ○ LONG, SLOW DISTANCE RUN
- ○ SPEED/TRACK WORKOUT
- ○ MY REGULAR RUN

WHERE
- ○ INDOOR
- ○ OUTDOOR

ROUTE

DISTANCE

TIME OF DAY/NIGHT

TIME

PACE

WEATHER

EFFORT
| 1 EASY | 2 EASY+ | 3 OK! | 4 OOF | 5 OMG |

COMMENTS

SUNDAY

STRETCHING/WARM-UP

GOAL(S) FOR WORKOUT

TYPE OF RUN
- ○ LONG, SLOW DISTANCE RUN
- ○ SPEED/TRACK WORKOUT
- ○ MY REGULAR RUN

WHERE
- ○ INDOOR
- ○ OUTDOOR

ROUTE

DISTANCE

TIME OF DAY/NIGHT

TIME

PACE

WEATHER

EFFORT
| 1 EASY | 2 EASY+ | 3 OK! | 4 OOF | 5 OMG |

COMMENTS

WEEK 14

BEGIN DATE

END DATE

TOTAL MILEAGE THIS WEEK

MONDAY

STRETCHING/WARM-UP

GOAL(S) FOR WORKOUT

TYPE OF RUN
- ○ LONG, SLOW DISTANCE RUN
- ○ SPEED/TRACK WORKOUT
- ○ MY REGULAR RUN

WHERE
- ○ INDOOR
- ○ OUTDOOR

ROUTE

DISTANCE

TIME OF DAY/NIGHT

TIME

PACE

WEATHER

EFFORT

| 1 EASY | 2 EASY+ | 3 OK! | 4 OOF | 5 OMG |

COMMENTS

TUESDAY

STRETCHING/WARM-UP

GOAL(S) FOR WORKOUT

TYPE OF RUN
- ○ LONG, SLOW DISTANCE RUN
- ○ SPEED/TRACK WORKOUT
- ○ MY REGULAR RUN

WHERE
- ○ INDOOR
- ○ OUTDOOR

ROUTE

DISTANCE

TIME OF DAY/NIGHT

TIME

PACE

WEATHER

EFFORT

| 1 EASY | 2 EASY+ | 3 OK! | 4 OOF | 5 OMG |

COMMENTS

WEDNESDAY

STRETCHING/WARM-UP

GOAL(S) FOR WORKOUT

TYPE OF RUN
- ○ LONG, SLOW DISTANCE RUN
- ○ SPEED/TRACK WORKOUT
- ○ MY REGULAR RUN

WHERE
- ○ INDOOR
- ○ OUTDOOR

ROUTE

DISTANCE

TIME OF DAY/NIGHT

TIME

PACE

WEATHER

EFFORT

| 1 EASY | 2 EASY+ | 3 OK! | 4 OOF | 5 OMG |

COMMENTS

THURSDAY

STRETCHING/WARM-UP

GOAL(S) FOR WORKOUT

TYPE OF RUN
- ○ LONG, SLOW DISTANCE RUN
- ○ SPEED/TRACK WORKOUT
- ○ MY REGULAR RUN

WHERE
- ○ INDOOR
- ○ OUTDOOR

ROUTE

DISTANCE

TIME OF DAY/NIGHT

TIME   PACE   WEATHER

EFFORT | 1 EASY | 2 EASY+ | 3 OK! | 4 OOF | 5 OMG |

COMMENTS

FRIDAY

STRETCHING/WARM-UP

GOAL(S) FOR WORKOUT

TYPE OF RUN
- ○ LONG, SLOW DISTANCE RUN
- ○ SPEED/TRACK WORKOUT
- ○ MY REGULAR RUN

WHERE
- ○ INDOOR
- ○ OUTDOOR

ROUTE

DISTANCE

TIME OF DAY/NIGHT

TIME   PACE   WEATHER

EFFORT | 1 EASY | 2 EASY+ | 3 OK! | 4 OOF | 5 OMG |

COMMENTS

SATURDAY

STRETCHING/WARM-UP

GOAL(S) FOR WORKOUT

TYPE OF RUN
- ○ LONG, SLOW DISTANCE RUN
- ○ SPEED/TRACK WORKOUT
- ○ MY REGULAR RUN

WHERE
- ○ INDOOR
- ○ OUTDOOR

ROUTE

DISTANCE

TIME OF DAY/NIGHT

TIME   PACE   WEATHER

EFFORT | 1 EASY | 2 EASY+ | 3 OK! | 4 OOF | 5 OMG |

COMMENTS

SUNDAY

STRETCHING/WARM-UP

GOAL(S) FOR WORKOUT

TYPE OF RUN
- ○ LONG, SLOW DISTANCE RUN
- ○ SPEED/TRACK WORKOUT
- ○ MY REGULAR RUN

WHERE
- ○ INDOOR
- ○ OUTDOOR

ROUTE

DISTANCE

TIME OF DAY/NIGHT

TIME   PACE   WEATHER

EFFORT | 1 EASY | 2 EASY+ | 3 OK! | 4 OOF | 5 OMG |

COMMENTS

WEEK 15

BEGIN DATE

END DATE

TOTAL MILEAGE THIS WEEK

MONDAY

STRETCHING/WARM-UP

GOAL(S) FOR WORKOUT

TYPE OF RUN
- ○ LONG, SLOW DISTANCE RUN
- ○ SPEED/TRACK WORKOUT
- ○ MY REGULAR RUN

WHERE
- ○ INDOOR
- ○ OUTDOOR

ROUTE

DISTANCE

TIME OF DAY/NIGHT

TIME

PACE

WEATHER

EFFORT

| 1 EASY | 2 EASY+ | 3 OK! | 4 OOF | 5 OMG |

COMMENTS

TUESDAY

STRETCHING/WARM-UP

GOAL(S) FOR WORKOUT

TYPE OF RUN
- ○ LONG, SLOW DISTANCE RUN
- ○ SPEED/TRACK WORKOUT
- ○ MY REGULAR RUN

WHERE
- ○ INDOOR
- ○ OUTDOOR

ROUTE

DISTANCE

TIME OF DAY/NIGHT

TIME

PACE

WEATHER

EFFORT

| 1 EASY | 2 EASY+ | 3 OK! | 4 OOF | 5 OMG |

COMMENTS

WEDNESDAY

STRETCHING/WARM-UP

GOAL(S) FOR WORKOUT

TYPE OF RUN
- ○ LONG, SLOW DISTANCE RUN
- ○ SPEED/TRACK WORKOUT
- ○ MY REGULAR RUN

WHERE
- ○ INDOOR
- ○ OUTDOOR

ROUTE

DISTANCE

TIME OF DAY/NIGHT

TIME

PACE

WEATHER

EFFORT

| 1 EASY | 2 EASY+ | 3 OK! | 4 OOF | 5 OMG |

COMMENTS

THURSDAY

STRETCHING/WARM-UP

GOAL(S) FOR WORKOUT

TYPE OF RUN
- ○ LONG, SLOW DISTANCE RUN
- ○ SPEED/TRACK WORKOUT
- ○ MY REGULAR RUN

WHERE
- ○ INDOOR
- ○ OUTDOOR

ROUTE

DISTANCE

TIME OF DAY/NIGHT

TIME   PACE   WEATHER

EFFORT | 1 EASY | 2 EASY+ | 3 OK! | 4 OOF | 5 OMG |

COMMENTS

FRIDAY

STRETCHING/WARM-UP

GOAL(S) FOR WORKOUT

TYPE OF RUN
- ○ LONG, SLOW DISTANCE RUN
- ○ SPEED/TRACK WORKOUT
- ○ MY REGULAR RUN

WHERE
- ○ INDOOR
- ○ OUTDOOR

ROUTE

DISTANCE

TIME OF DAY/NIGHT

TIME   PACE   WEATHER

EFFORT | 1 EASY | 2 EASY+ | 3 OK! | 4 OOF | 5 OMG |

COMMENTS

SATURDAY

STRETCHING/WARM-UP

GOAL(S) FOR WORKOUT

TYPE OF RUN
- ○ LONG, SLOW DISTANCE RUN
- ○ SPEED/TRACK WORKOUT
- ○ MY REGULAR RUN

WHERE
- ○ INDOOR
- ○ OUTDOOR

ROUTE

DISTANCE

TIME OF DAY/NIGHT

TIME   PACE   WEATHER

EFFORT | 1 EASY | 2 EASY+ | 3 OK! | 4 OOF | 5 OMG |

COMMENTS

SUNDAY

STRETCHING/WARM-UP

GOAL(S) FOR WORKOUT

TYPE OF RUN
- ○ LONG, SLOW DISTANCE RUN
- ○ SPEED/TRACK WORKOUT
- ○ MY REGULAR RUN

WHERE
- ○ INDOOR
- ○ OUTDOOR

ROUTE

DISTANCE

TIME OF DAY/NIGHT

TIME   PACE   WEATHER

EFFORT | 1 EASY | 2 EASY+ | 3 OK! | 4 OOF | 5 OMG |

COMMENTS

WEEK 16

BEGIN DATE	END DATE

TOTAL MILEAGE THIS WEEK

MONDAY

STRETCHING/WARM-UP

GOAL(S) FOR WORKOUT

TYPE OF RUN
- ○ LONG, SLOW DISTANCE RUN
- ○ SPEED/TRACK WORKOUT
- ○ MY REGULAR RUN

WHERE
- ○ INDOOR
- ○ OUTDOOR

ROUTE

DISTANCE

TIME OF DAY/NIGHT

TIME   PACE   WEATHER

EFFORT

1 EASY	2 EASY+	3 OK!	4 OOF	5 OMG

COMMENTS

TUESDAY

STRETCHING/WARM-UP

GOAL(S) FOR WORKOUT

TYPE OF RUN
- ○ LONG, SLOW DISTANCE RUN
- ○ SPEED/TRACK WORKOUT
- ○ MY REGULAR RUN

WHERE
- ○ INDOOR
- ○ OUTDOOR

ROUTE

DISTANCE

TIME OF DAY/NIGHT

TIME   PACE   WEATHER

EFFORT

1 EASY	2 EASY+	3 OK!	4 OOF	5 OMG

COMMENTS

WEDNESDAY

STRETCHING/WARM-UP

GOAL(S) FOR WORKOUT

TYPE OF RUN
- ○ LONG, SLOW DISTANCE RUN
- ○ SPEED/TRACK WORKOUT
- ○ MY REGULAR RUN

WHERE
- ○ INDOOR
- ○ OUTDOOR

ROUTE

DISTANCE

TIME OF DAY/NIGHT

TIME   PACE   WEATHER

EFFORT

1 EASY	2 EASY+	3 OK!	4 OOF	5 OMG

COMMENTS

THURSDAY

STRETCHING/WARM-UP	DISTANCE	TIME OF DAY/NIGHT

GOAL(S) FOR WORKOUT	TIME	PACE	WEATHER

TYPE OF RUN
- ○ LONG, SLOW DISTANCE RUN
- ○ SPEED/TRACK WORKOUT
- ○ MY REGULAR RUN

WHERE
- ○ INDOOR
- ○ OUTDOOR

EFFORT | 1 EASY | 2 EASY+ | 3 OK! | 4 OOF | 5 OMG |

COMMENTS

ROUTE

FRIDAY

STRETCHING/WARM-UP	DISTANCE	TIME OF DAY/NIGHT

GOAL(S) FOR WORKOUT	TIME	PACE	WEATHER

TYPE OF RUN
- ○ LONG, SLOW DISTANCE RUN
- ○ SPEED/TRACK WORKOUT
- ○ MY REGULAR RUN

WHERE
- ○ INDOOR
- ○ OUTDOOR

EFFORT | 1 EASY | 2 EASY+ | 3 OK! | 4 OOF | 5 OMG |

COMMENTS

ROUTE

SATURDAY

STRETCHING/WARM-UP	DISTANCE	TIME OF DAY/NIGHT

GOAL(S) FOR WORKOUT	TIME	PACE	WEATHER

TYPE OF RUN
- ○ LONG, SLOW DISTANCE RUN
- ○ SPEED/TRACK WORKOUT
- ○ MY REGULAR RUN

WHERE
- ○ INDOOR
- ○ OUTDOOR

EFFORT | 1 EASY | 2 EASY+ | 3 OK! | 4 OOF | 5 OMG |

COMMENTS

ROUTE

SUNDAY

STRETCHING/WARM-UP	DISTANCE	TIME OF DAY/NIGHT

GOAL(S) FOR WORKOUT	TIME	PACE	WEATHER

TYPE OF RUN
- ○ LONG, SLOW DISTANCE RUN
- ○ SPEED/TRACK WORKOUT
- ○ MY REGULAR RUN

WHERE
- ○ INDOOR
- ○ OUTDOOR

EFFORT | 1 EASY | 2 EASY+ | 3 OK! | 4 OOF | 5 OMG |

COMMENTS

ROUTE

WEEK 17

BEGIN DATE

END DATE

TOTAL MILEAGE THIS WEEK

MONDAY

STRETCHING/WARM-UP

GOAL(S) FOR WORKOUT

TYPE OF RUN
- ○ LONG, SLOW DISTANCE RUN
- ○ SPEED/TRACK WORKOUT
- ○ MY REGULAR RUN

WHERE
- ○ INDOOR
- ○ OUTDOOR

ROUTE

DISTANCE

TIME OF DAY/NIGHT

TIME

PACE

WEATHER

EFFORT

| 1 EASY | 2 EASY+ | 3 OK! | 4 OOF | 5 OMG |

COMMENTS

TUESDAY

STRETCHING/WARM-UP

GOAL(S) FOR WORKOUT

TYPE OF RUN
- ○ LONG, SLOW DISTANCE RUN
- ○ SPEED/TRACK WORKOUT
- ○ MY REGULAR RUN

WHERE
- ○ INDOOR
- ○ OUTDOOR

ROUTE

DISTANCE

TIME OF DAY/NIGHT

TIME

PACE

WEATHER

EFFORT

| 1 EASY | 2 EASY+ | 3 OK! | 4 OOF | 5 OMG |

COMMENTS

WEDNESDAY

STRETCHING/WARM-UP

GOAL(S) FOR WORKOUT

TYPE OF RUN
- ○ LONG, SLOW DISTANCE RUN
- ○ SPEED/TRACK WORKOUT
- ○ MY REGULAR RUN

WHERE
- ○ INDOOR
- ○ OUTDOOR

ROUTE

DISTANCE

TIME OF DAY/NIGHT

TIME

PACE

WEATHER

EFFORT

| 1 EASY | 2 EASY+ | 3 OK! | 4 OOF | 5 OMG |

COMMENTS

THURSDAY

STRETCHING/WARM-UP

GOAL(S) FOR WORKOUT

TYPE OF RUN
- ○ LONG, SLOW DISTANCE RUN
- ○ SPEED/TRACK WORKOUT
- ○ MY REGULAR RUN

WHERE
- ○ INDOOR
- ○ OUTDOOR

ROUTE

DISTANCE

TIME OF DAY/NIGHT

TIME   PACE   WEATHER

EFFORT

| 1 EASY | 2 EASY+ | 3 OK! | 4 OOF | 5 OMG |

COMMENTS

FRIDAY

STRETCHING/WARM-UP

GOAL(S) FOR WORKOUT

TYPE OF RUN
- ○ LONG, SLOW DISTANCE RUN
- ○ SPEED/TRACK WORKOUT
- ○ MY REGULAR RUN

WHERE
- ○ INDOOR
- ○ OUTDOOR

ROUTE

DISTANCE

TIME OF DAY/NIGHT

TIME   PACE   WEATHER

EFFORT

| 1 EASY | 2 EASY+ | 3 OK! | 4 OOF | 5 OMG |

COMMENTS

SATURDAY

STRETCHING/WARM-UP

GOAL(S) FOR WORKOUT

TYPE OF RUN
- ○ LONG, SLOW DISTANCE RUN
- ○ SPEED/TRACK WORKOUT
- ○ MY REGULAR RUN

WHERE
- ○ INDOOR
- ○ OUTDOOR

ROUTE

DISTANCE

TIME OF DAY/NIGHT

TIME   PACE   WEATHER

EFFORT

| 1 EASY | 2 EASY+ | 3 OK! | 4 OOF | 5 OMG |

COMMENTS

SUNDAY

STRETCHING/WARM-UP

GOAL(S) FOR WORKOUT

TYPE OF RUN
- ○ LONG, SLOW DISTANCE RUN
- ○ SPEED/TRACK WORKOUT
- ○ MY REGULAR RUN

WHERE
- ○ INDOOR
- ○ OUTDOOR

ROUTE

DISTANCE

TIME OF DAY/NIGHT

TIME   PACE   WEATHER

EFFORT

| 1 EASY | 2 EASY+ | 3 OK! | 4 OOF | 5 OMG |

COMMENTS

WEEK 18

BEGIN DATE	END DATE

TOTAL MILEAGE THIS WEEK

MONDAY

STRETCHING/WARM-UP

DISTANCE

TIME OF DAY/NIGHT

GOAL(S) FOR WORKOUT

TIME

PACE

WEATHER

TYPE OF RUN
○ LONG, SLOW DISTANCE RUN
○ SPEED/TRACK WORKOUT
○ MY REGULAR RUN

WHERE
○ INDOOR
○ OUTDOOR

EFFORT

1 EASY	2 EASY+	3 OK!	4 OOF	5 OMG

COMMENTS

ROUTE

TUESDAY

STRETCHING/WARM-UP

DISTANCE

TIME OF DAY/NIGHT

GOAL(S) FOR WORKOUT

TIME

PACE

WEATHER

TYPE OF RUN
○ LONG, SLOW DISTANCE RUN
○ SPEED/TRACK WORKOUT
○ MY REGULAR RUN

WHERE
○ INDOOR
○ OUTDOOR

EFFORT

1 EASY	2 EASY+	3 OK!	4 OOF	5 OMG

COMMENTS

ROUTE

WEDNESDAY

STRETCHING/WARM-UP

DISTANCE

TIME OF DAY/NIGHT

GOAL(S) FOR WORKOUT

TIME

PACE

WEATHER

TYPE OF RUN
○ LONG, SLOW DISTANCE RUN
○ SPEED/TRACK WORKOUT
○ MY REGULAR RUN

WHERE
○ INDOOR
○ OUTDOOR

EFFORT

1 EASY	2 EASY+	3 OK!	4 OOF	5 OMG

COMMENTS

ROUTE

THURSDAY

STRETCHING/WARM-UP

GOAL(S) FOR WORKOUT

TYPE OF RUN
○ LONG, SLOW DISTANCE RUN
○ SPEED/TRACK WORKOUT
○ MY REGULAR RUN

WHERE
○ INDOOR
○ OUTDOOR

ROUTE

DISTANCE

TIME OF DAY/NIGHT

TIME   PACE   WEATHER

EFFORT | 1 EASY | 2 EASY+ | 3 OK! | 4 OOF | 5 OMG |

COMMENTS

FRIDAY

STRETCHING/WARM-UP

GOAL(S) FOR WORKOUT

TYPE OF RUN
○ LONG, SLOW DISTANCE RUN
○ SPEED/TRACK WORKOUT
○ MY REGULAR RUN

WHERE
○ INDOOR
○ OUTDOOR

ROUTE

DISTANCE

TIME OF DAY/NIGHT

TIME   PACE   WEATHER

EFFORT | 1 EASY | 2 EASY+ | 3 OK! | 4 OOF | 5 OMG |

COMMENTS

SATURDAY

STRETCHING/WARM-UP

GOAL(S) FOR WORKOUT

TYPE OF RUN
○ LONG, SLOW DISTANCE RUN
○ SPEED/TRACK WORKOUT
○ MY REGULAR RUN

WHERE
○ INDOOR
○ OUTDOOR

ROUTE

DISTANCE

TIME OF DAY/NIGHT

TIME   PACE   WEATHER

EFFORT | 1 EASY | 2 EASY+ | 3 OK! | 4 OOF | 5 OMG |

COMMENTS

SUNDAY

STRETCHING/WARM-UP

GOAL(S) FOR WORKOUT

TYPE OF RUN
○ LONG, SLOW DISTANCE RUN
○ SPEED/TRACK WORKOUT
○ MY REGULAR RUN

WHERE
○ INDOOR
○ OUTDOOR

ROUTE

DISTANCE

TIME OF DAY/NIGHT

TIME   PACE   WEATHER

EFFORT | 1 EASY | 2 EASY+ | 3 OK! | 4 OOF | 5 OMG |

COMMENTS

WEEK 19

BEGIN DATE

END DATE

TOTAL MILEAGE THIS WEEK

MONDAY

STRETCHING/WARM-UP

GOAL(S) FOR WORKOUT

TYPE OF RUN
- ○ LONG, SLOW DISTANCE RUN
- ○ SPEED/TRACK WORKOUT
- ○ MY REGULAR RUN

WHERE
- ○ INDOOR
- ○ OUTDOOR

ROUTE

DISTANCE

TIME OF DAY/NIGHT

TIME   PACE   WEATHER

EFFORT

| 1 EASY | 2 EASY+ | 3 OK! | 4 OOF | 5 OMG |

COMMENTS

TUESDAY

STRETCHING/WARM-UP

GOAL(S) FOR WORKOUT

TYPE OF RUN
- ○ LONG, SLOW DISTANCE RUN
- ○ SPEED/TRACK WORKOUT
- ○ MY REGULAR RUN

WHERE
- ○ INDOOR
- ○ OUTDOOR

ROUTE

DISTANCE

TIME OF DAY/NIGHT

TIME   PACE   WEATHER

EFFORT

| 1 EASY | 2 EASY+ | 3 OK! | 4 OOF | 5 OMG |

COMMENTS

WEDNESDAY

STRETCHING/WARM-UP

GOAL(S) FOR WORKOUT

TYPE OF RUN
- ○ LONG, SLOW DISTANCE RUN
- ○ SPEED/TRACK WORKOUT
- ○ MY REGULAR RUN

WHERE
- ○ INDOOR
- ○ OUTDOOR

ROUTE

DISTANCE

TIME OF DAY/NIGHT

TIME   PACE   WEATHER

EFFORT

| 1 EASY | 2 EASY+ | 3 OK! | 4 OOF | 5 OMG |

COMMENTS

THURSDAY

STRETCHING/WARM-UP		DISTANCE		TIME OF DAY/NIGHT

GOAL(S) FOR WORKOUT

TIME	PACE	WEATHER

TYPE OF RUN
- ○ LONG, SLOW DISTANCE RUN
- ○ SPEED/TRACK WORKOUT
- ○ MY REGULAR RUN

WHERE
- ○ INDOOR
- ○ OUTDOOR

EFFORT

1 EASY	2 EASY+	3 OK!	4 OOF	5 OMG

COMMENTS

ROUTE

FRIDAY

STRETCHING/WARM-UP		DISTANCE		TIME OF DAY/NIGHT

GOAL(S) FOR WORKOUT

TIME	PACE	WEATHER

TYPE OF RUN
- ○ LONG, SLOW DISTANCE RUN
- ○ SPEED/TRACK WORKOUT
- ○ MY REGULAR RUN

WHERE
- ○ INDOOR
- ○ OUTDOOR

EFFORT

1 EASY	2 EASY+	3 OK!	4 OOF	5 OMG

COMMENTS

ROUTE

SATURDAY

STRETCHING/WARM-UP		DISTANCE		TIME OF DAY/NIGHT

GOAL(S) FOR WORKOUT

TIME	PACE	WEATHER

TYPE OF RUN
- ○ LONG, SLOW DISTANCE RUN
- ○ SPEED/TRACK WORKOUT
- ○ MY REGULAR RUN

WHERE
- ○ INDOOR
- ○ OUTDOOR

EFFORT

1 EASY	2 EASY+	3 OK!	4 OOF	5 OMG

COMMENTS

ROUTE

SUNDAY

STRETCHING/WARM-UP		DISTANCE		TIME OF DAY/NIGHT

GOAL(S) FOR WORKOUT

TIME	PACE	WEATHER

TYPE OF RUN
- ○ LONG, SLOW DISTANCE RUN
- ○ SPEED/TRACK WORKOUT
- ○ MY REGULAR RUN

WHERE
- ○ INDOOR
- ○ OUTDOOR

EFFORT

1 EASY	2 EASY+	3 OK!	4 OOF	5 OMG

COMMENTS

ROUTE

WEEK 20

BEGIN DATE

END DATE

TOTAL MILEAGE THIS WEEK

MONDAY

STRETCHING/WARM-UP

GOAL(S) FOR WORKOUT

TYPE OF RUN
- ○ LONG, SLOW DISTANCE RUN
- ○ SPEED/TRACK WORKOUT
- ○ MY REGULAR RUN

WHERE
- ○ INDOOR
- ○ OUTDOOR

ROUTE

DISTANCE

TIME OF DAY/NIGHT

TIME

PACE

WEATHER

EFFORT

| 1 EASY | 2 EASY+ | 3 OK! | 4 OOF | 5 OMG |

COMMENTS

TUESDAY

STRETCHING/WARM-UP

GOAL(S) FOR WORKOUT

TYPE OF RUN
- ○ LONG, SLOW DISTANCE RUN
- ○ SPEED/TRACK WORKOUT
- ○ MY REGULAR RUN

WHERE
- ○ INDOOR
- ○ OUTDOOR

ROUTE

DISTANCE

TIME OF DAY/NIGHT

TIME

PACE

WEATHER

EFFORT

| 1 EASY | 2 EASY+ | 3 OK! | 4 OOF | 5 OMG |

COMMENTS

WEDNESDAY

STRETCHING/WARM-UP

GOAL(S) FOR WORKOUT

TYPE OF RUN
- ○ LONG, SLOW DISTANCE RUN
- ○ SPEED/TRACK WORKOUT
- ○ MY REGULAR RUN

WHERE
- ○ INDOOR
- ○ OUTDOOR

ROUTE

DISTANCE

TIME OF DAY/NIGHT

TIME

PACE

WEATHER

EFFORT

| 1 EASY | 2 EASY+ | 3 OK! | 4 OOF | 5 OMG |

COMMENTS

THURSDAY

STRETCHING/WARM-UP

DISTANCE

TIME OF DAY/NIGHT

GOAL(S) FOR WORKOUT

TIME

PACE

WEATHER

TYPE OF RUN
- ○ LONG, SLOW DISTANCE RUN
- ○ SPEED/TRACK WORKOUT
- ○ MY REGULAR RUN

WHERE
- ○ INDOOR
- ○ OUTDOOR

EFFORT

| 1 EASY | 2 EASY+ | 3 OK! | 4 OOF | 5 OMG |

COMMENTS

ROUTE

FRIDAY

STRETCHING/WARM-UP

DISTANCE

TIME OF DAY/NIGHT

GOAL(S) FOR WORKOUT

TIME

PACE

WEATHER

TYPE OF RUN
- ○ LONG, SLOW DISTANCE RUN
- ○ SPEED/TRACK WORKOUT
- ○ MY REGULAR RUN

WHERE
- ○ INDOOR
- ○ OUTDOOR

EFFORT

| 1 EASY | 2 EASY+ | 3 OK! | 4 OOF | 5 OMG |

COMMENTS

ROUTE

SATURDAY

STRETCHING/WARM-UP

DISTANCE

TIME OF DAY/NIGHT

GOAL(S) FOR WORKOUT

TIME

PACE

WEATHER

TYPE OF RUN
- ○ LONG, SLOW DISTANCE RUN
- ○ SPEED/TRACK WORKOUT
- ○ MY REGULAR RUN

WHERE
- ○ INDOOR
- ○ OUTDOOR

EFFORT

| 1 EASY | 2 EASY+ | 3 OK! | 4 OOF | 5 OMG |

COMMENTS

ROUTE

SUNDAY

STRETCHING/WARM-UP

DISTANCE

TIME OF DAY/NIGHT

GOAL(S) FOR WORKOUT

TIME

PACE

WEATHER

TYPE OF RUN
- ○ LONG, SLOW DISTANCE RUN
- ○ SPEED/TRACK WORKOUT
- ○ MY REGULAR RUN

WHERE
- ○ INDOOR
- ○ OUTDOOR

EFFORT

| 1 EASY | 2 EASY+ | 3 OK! | 4 OOF | 5 OMG |

COMMENTS

ROUTE

WEEK 21

BEGIN DATE

END DATE

TOTAL MILEAGE THIS WEEK

MONDAY

STRETCHING/WARM-UP

GOAL(S) FOR WORKOUT

TYPE OF RUN
- ○ LONG, SLOW DISTANCE RUN
- ○ SPEED/TRACK WORKOUT
- ○ MY REGULAR RUN

WHERE
- ○ INDOOR
- ○ OUTDOOR

ROUTE

DISTANCE

TIME OF DAY/NIGHT

TIME   PACE   WEATHER

EFFORT

| 1 EASY | 2 EASY+ | 3 OK! | 4 OOF | 5 OMG |

COMMENTS

TUESDAY

STRETCHING/WARM-UP

GOAL(S) FOR WORKOUT

TYPE OF RUN
- ○ LONG, SLOW DISTANCE RUN
- ○ SPEED/TRACK WORKOUT
- ○ MY REGULAR RUN

WHERE
- ○ INDOOR
- ○ OUTDOOR

ROUTE

DISTANCE

TIME OF DAY/NIGHT

TIME   PACE   WEATHER

EFFORT

| 1 EASY | 2 EASY+ | 3 OK! | 4 OOF | 5 OMG |

COMMENTS

WEDNESDAY

STRETCHING/WARM-UP

GOAL(S) FOR WORKOUT

TYPE OF RUN
- ○ LONG, SLOW DISTANCE RUN
- ○ SPEED/TRACK WORKOUT
- ○ MY REGULAR RUN

WHERE
- ○ INDOOR
- ○ OUTDOOR

ROUTE

DISTANCE

TIME OF DAY/NIGHT

TIME   PACE   WEATHER

EFFORT

| 1 EASY | 2 EASY+ | 3 OK! | 4 OOF | 5 OMG |

COMMENTS

THURSDAY

STRETCHING/WARM-UP

DISTANCE

TIME OF DAY/NIGHT

GOAL(S) FOR WORKOUT

TIME   PACE   WEATHER

TYPE OF RUN
○ LONG, SLOW DISTANCE RUN
○ SPEED/TRACK WORKOUT
○ MY REGULAR RUN

WHERE
○ INDOOR
○ OUTDOOR

EFFORT

1 EASY	2 EASY+	3 OK!	4 OOF	5 OMG

COMMENTS

ROUTE

FRIDAY

STRETCHING/WARM-UP

DISTANCE

TIME OF DAY/NIGHT

GOAL(S) FOR WORKOUT

TIME   PACE   WEATHER

TYPE OF RUN
○ LONG, SLOW DISTANCE RUN
○ SPEED/TRACK WORKOUT
○ MY REGULAR RUN

WHERE
○ INDOOR
○ OUTDOOR

EFFORT

1 EASY	2 EASY+	3 OK!	4 OOF	5 OMG

COMMENTS

ROUTE

SATURDAY

STRETCHING/WARM-UP

DISTANCE

TIME OF DAY/NIGHT

GOAL(S) FOR WORKOUT

TIME   PACE   WEATHER

TYPE OF RUN
○ LONG, SLOW DISTANCE RUN
○ SPEED/TRACK WORKOUT
○ MY REGULAR RUN

WHERE
○ INDOOR
○ OUTDOOR

EFFORT

1 EASY	2 EASY+	3 OK!	4 OOF	5 OMG

COMMENTS

ROUTE

SUNDAY

STRETCHING/WARM-UP

DISTANCE

TIME OF DAY/NIGHT

GOAL(S) FOR WORKOUT

TIME   PACE   WEATHER

TYPE OF RUN
○ LONG, SLOW DISTANCE RUN
○ SPEED/TRACK WORKOUT
○ MY REGULAR RUN

WHERE
○ INDOOR
○ OUTDOOR

EFFORT

1 EASY	2 EASY+	3 OK!	4 OOF	5 OMG

COMMENTS

ROUTE

WEEK 22

BEGIN DATE

END DATE

TOTAL MILEAGE THIS WEEK

MONDAY

STRETCHING/WARM-UP

DISTANCE

TIME OF DAY/NIGHT

GOAL(S) FOR WORKOUT

TIME

PACE

WEATHER

TYPE OF RUN
- ○ LONG, SLOW DISTANCE RUN
- ○ SPEED/TRACK WORKOUT
- ○ MY REGULAR RUN

WHERE
- ○ INDOOR
- ○ OUTDOOR

EFFORT

| 1 EASY | 2 EASY+ | 3 OK! | 4 OOF | 5 OMG |

COMMENTS

ROUTE

TUESDAY

STRETCHING/WARM-UP

DISTANCE

TIME OF DAY/NIGHT

GOAL(S) FOR WORKOUT

TIME

PACE

WEATHER

TYPE OF RUN
- ○ LONG, SLOW DISTANCE RUN
- ○ SPEED/TRACK WORKOUT
- ○ MY REGULAR RUN

WHERE
- ○ INDOOR
- ○ OUTDOOR

EFFORT

| 1 EASY | 2 EASY+ | 3 OK! | 4 OOF | 5 OMG |

COMMENTS

ROUTE

WEDNESDAY

STRETCHING/WARM-UP

DISTANCE

TIME OF DAY/NIGHT

GOAL(S) FOR WORKOUT

TIME

PACE

WEATHER

TYPE OF RUN
- ○ LONG, SLOW DISTANCE RUN
- ○ SPEED/TRACK WORKOUT
- ○ MY REGULAR RUN

WHERE
- ○ INDOOR
- ○ OUTDOOR

EFFORT

| 1 EASY | 2 EASY+ | 3 OK! | 4 OOF | 5 OMG |

COMMENTS

ROUTE

THURSDAY

STRETCHING/WARM-UP

GOAL(S) FOR WORKOUT

TYPE OF RUN
- ○ LONG, SLOW DISTANCE RUN
- ○ SPEED/TRACK WORKOUT
- ○ MY REGULAR RUN

WHERE
- ○ INDOOR
- ○ OUTDOOR

ROUTE

DISTANCE

TIME OF DAY/NIGHT

TIME

PACE

WEATHER

EFFORT
| 1 EASY | 2 EASY+ | 3 OK! | 4 OOF | 5 OMG |

COMMENTS

FRIDAY

STRETCHING/WARM-UP

GOAL(S) FOR WORKOUT

TYPE OF RUN
- ○ LONG, SLOW DISTANCE RUN
- ○ SPEED/TRACK WORKOUT
- ○ MY REGULAR RUN

WHERE
- ○ INDOOR
- ○ OUTDOOR

ROUTE

DISTANCE

TIME OF DAY/NIGHT

TIME

PACE

WEATHER

EFFORT
| 1 EASY | 2 EASY+ | 3 OK! | 4 OOF | 5 OMG |

COMMENTS

SATURDAY

STRETCHING/WARM-UP

GOAL(S) FOR WORKOUT

TYPE OF RUN
- ○ LONG, SLOW DISTANCE RUN
- ○ SPEED/TRACK WORKOUT
- ○ MY REGULAR RUN

WHERE
- ○ INDOOR
- ○ OUTDOOR

ROUTE

DISTANCE

TIME OF DAY/NIGHT

TIME

PACE

WEATHER

EFFORT
| 1 EASY | 2 EASY+ | 3 OK! | 4 OOF | 5 OMG |

COMMENTS

SUNDAY

STRETCHING/WARM-UP

GOAL(S) FOR WORKOUT

TYPE OF RUN
- ○ LONG, SLOW DISTANCE RUN
- ○ SPEED/TRACK WORKOUT
- ○ MY REGULAR RUN

WHERE
- ○ INDOOR
- ○ OUTDOOR

ROUTE

DISTANCE

TIME OF DAY/NIGHT

TIME

PACE

WEATHER

EFFORT
| 1 EASY | 2 EASY+ | 3 OK! | 4 OOF | 5 OMG |

COMMENTS

WEEK 23

BEGIN DATE

END DATE

TOTAL MILEAGE THIS WEEK

MONDAY

STRETCHING/WARM-UP

DISTANCE

TIME OF DAY/NIGHT

GOAL(S) FOR WORKOUT

TIME

PACE

WEATHER

TYPE OF RUN
- ○ LONG, SLOW DISTANCE RUN
- ○ SPEED/TRACK WORKOUT
- ○ MY REGULAR RUN

WHERE
- ○ INDOOR
- ○ OUTDOOR

EFFORT

| 1 EASY | 2 EASY+ | 3 OK! | 4 OOF | 5 OMG |

COMMENTS

ROUTE

TUESDAY

STRETCHING/WARM-UP

DISTANCE

TIME OF DAY/NIGHT

GOAL(S) FOR WORKOUT

TIME

PACE

WEATHER

TYPE OF RUN
- ○ LONG, SLOW DISTANCE RUN
- ○ SPEED/TRACK WORKOUT
- ○ MY REGULAR RUN

WHERE
- ○ INDOOR
- ○ OUTDOOR

EFFORT

| 1 EASY | 2 EASY+ | 3 OK! | 4 OOF | 5 OMG |

COMMENTS

ROUTE

WEDNESDAY

STRETCHING/WARM-UP

DISTANCE

TIME OF DAY/NIGHT

GOAL(S) FOR WORKOUT

TIME

PACE

WEATHER

TYPE OF RUN
- ○ LONG, SLOW DISTANCE RUN
- ○ SPEED/TRACK WORKOUT
- ○ MY REGULAR RUN

WHERE
- ○ INDOOR
- ○ OUTDOOR

EFFORT

| 1 EASY | 2 EASY+ | 3 OK! | 4 OOF | 5 OMG |

COMMENTS

ROUTE

THURSDAY

STRETCHING/WARM-UP

GOAL(S) FOR WORKOUT

TYPE OF RUN
- ○ LONG, SLOW DISTANCE RUN
- ○ SPEED/TRACK WORKOUT
- ○ MY REGULAR RUN

WHERE
- ○ INDOOR
- ○ OUTDOOR

ROUTE

DISTANCE

TIME OF DAY/NIGHT

TIME   **PACE**   **WEATHER**

EFFORT

1 EASY	2 EASY+	3 OK!	4 OOF	5 OMG

COMMENTS

FRIDAY

STRETCHING/WARM-UP

GOAL(S) FOR WORKOUT

TYPE OF RUN
- ○ LONG, SLOW DISTANCE RUN
- ○ SPEED/TRACK WORKOUT
- ○ MY REGULAR RUN

WHERE
- ○ INDOOR
- ○ OUTDOOR

ROUTE

DISTANCE

TIME OF DAY/NIGHT

TIME   **PACE**   **WEATHER**

EFFORT

1 EASY	2 EASY+	3 OK!	4 OOF	5 OMG

COMMENTS

SATURDAY

STRETCHING/WARM-UP

GOAL(S) FOR WORKOUT

TYPE OF RUN
- ○ LONG, SLOW DISTANCE RUN
- ○ SPEED/TRACK WORKOUT
- ○ MY REGULAR RUN

WHERE
- ○ INDOOR
- ○ OUTDOOR

ROUTE

DISTANCE

TIME OF DAY/NIGHT

TIME   **PACE**   **WEATHER**

EFFORT

1 EASY	2 EASY+	3 OK!	4 OOF	5 OMG

COMMENTS

SUNDAY

STRETCHING/WARM-UP

GOAL(S) FOR WORKOUT

TYPE OF RUN
- ○ LONG, SLOW DISTANCE RUN
- ○ SPEED/TRACK WORKOUT
- ○ MY REGULAR RUN

WHERE
- ○ INDOOR
- ○ OUTDOOR

ROUTE

DISTANCE

TIME OF DAY/NIGHT

TIME   **PACE**   **WEATHER**

EFFORT

1 EASY	2 EASY+	3 OK!	4 OOF	5 OMG

COMMENTS

WEEK 24

BEGIN DATE

END DATE

TOTAL MILEAGE THIS WEEK

MONDAY

STRETCHING/WARM-UP

DISTANCE

TIME OF DAY/NIGHT

GOAL(S) FOR WORKOUT

TIME

PACE

WEATHER

TYPE OF RUN
- ○ LONG, SLOW DISTANCE RUN
- ○ SPEED/TRACK WORKOUT
- ○ MY REGULAR RUN

WHERE
- ○ INDOOR
- ○ OUTDOOR

EFFORT

| 1 EASY | 2 EASY+ | 3 OK! | 4 OOF | 5 OMG |

COMMENTS

ROUTE

TUESDAY

STRETCHING/WARM-UP

DISTANCE

TIME OF DAY/NIGHT

GOAL(S) FOR WORKOUT

TIME

PACE

WEATHER

TYPE OF RUN
- ○ LONG, SLOW DISTANCE RUN
- ○ SPEED/TRACK WORKOUT
- ○ MY REGULAR RUN

WHERE
- ○ INDOOR
- ○ OUTDOOR

EFFORT

| 1 EASY | 2 EASY+ | 3 OK! | 4 OOF | 5 OMG |

COMMENTS

ROUTE

WEDNESDAY

STRETCHING/WARM-UP

DISTANCE

TIME OF DAY/NIGHT

GOAL(S) FOR WORKOUT

TIME

PACE

WEATHER

TYPE OF RUN
- ○ LONG, SLOW DISTANCE RUN
- ○ SPEED/TRACK WORKOUT
- ○ MY REGULAR RUN

WHERE
- ○ INDOOR
- ○ OUTDOOR

EFFORT

| 1 EASY | 2 EASY+ | 3 OK! | 4 OOF | 5 OMG |

COMMENTS

ROUTE

THURSDAY

| STRETCHING/WARM-UP | | | DISTANCE | | | TIME OF DAY/NIGHT |

GOAL(S) FOR WORKOUT

TIME   PACE   WEATHER

TYPE OF RUN
○ LONG, SLOW DISTANCE RUN
○ SPEED/TRACK WORKOUT
○ MY REGULAR RUN

WHERE
○ INDOOR
○ OUTDOOR

EFFORT | 1 EASY | 2 EASY+ | 3 OK! | 4 OOF | 5 OMG |

COMMENTS

ROUTE

FRIDAY

STRETCHING/WARM-UP

DISTANCE   TIME OF DAY/NIGHT

GOAL(S) FOR WORKOUT

TIME   PACE   WEATHER

TYPE OF RUN
○ LONG, SLOW DISTANCE RUN
○ SPEED/TRACK WORKOUT
○ MY REGULAR RUN

WHERE
○ INDOOR
○ OUTDOOR

EFFORT | 1 EASY | 2 EASY+ | 3 OK! | 4 OOF | 5 OMG |

COMMENTS

ROUTE

SATURDAY

STRETCHING/WARM-UP

DISTANCE   TIME OF DAY/NIGHT

GOAL(S) FOR WORKOUT

TIME   PACE   WEATHER

TYPE OF RUN
○ LONG, SLOW DISTANCE RUN
○ SPEED/TRACK WORKOUT
○ MY REGULAR RUN

WHERE
○ INDOOR
○ OUTDOOR

EFFORT | 1 EASY | 2 EASY+ | 3 OK! | 4 OOF | 5 OMG |

COMMENTS

ROUTE

SUNDAY

STRETCHING/WARM-UP

DISTANCE   TIME OF DAY/NIGHT

GOAL(S) FOR WORKOUT

TIME   PACE   WEATHER

TYPE OF RUN
○ LONG, SLOW DISTANCE RUN
○ SPEED/TRACK WORKOUT
○ MY REGULAR RUN

WHERE
○ INDOOR
○ OUTDOOR

EFFORT | 1 EASY | 2 EASY+ | 3 OK! | 4 OOF | 5 OMG |

COMMENTS

ROUTE

WEEK 25

BEGIN DATE

END DATE

TOTAL MILEAGE THIS WEEK

MONDAY

STRETCHING/WARM-UP

GOAL(S) FOR WORKOUT

TYPE OF RUN
- ○ LONG, SLOW DISTANCE RUN
- ○ SPEED/TRACK WORKOUT
- ○ MY REGULAR RUN

WHERE
- ○ INDOOR
- ○ OUTDOOR

ROUTE

DISTANCE

TIME OF DAY/NIGHT

TIME

PACE

WEATHER

EFFORT

| 1 EASY | 2 EASY+ | 3 OK! | 4 OOF | 5 OMG |

COMMENTS

TUESDAY

STRETCHING/WARM-UP

GOAL(S) FOR WORKOUT

TYPE OF RUN
- ○ LONG, SLOW DISTANCE RUN
- ○ SPEED/TRACK WORKOUT
- ○ MY REGULAR RUN

WHERE
- ○ INDOOR
- ○ OUTDOOR

ROUTE

DISTANCE

TIME OF DAY/NIGHT

TIME

PACE

WEATHER

EFFORT

| 1 EASY | 2 EASY+ | 3 OK! | 4 OOF | 5 OMG |

COMMENTS

WEDNESDAY

STRETCHING/WARM-UP

GOAL(S) FOR WORKOUT

TYPE OF RUN
- ○ LONG, SLOW DISTANCE RUN
- ○ SPEED/TRACK WORKOUT
- ○ MY REGULAR RUN

WHERE
- ○ INDOOR
- ○ OUTDOOR

ROUTE

DISTANCE

TIME OF DAY/NIGHT

TIME

PACE

WEATHER

EFFORT

| 1 EASY | 2 EASY+ | 3 OK! | 4 OOF | 5 OMG |

COMMENTS

THURSDAY

STRETCHING/WARM-UP

GOAL(S) FOR WORKOUT

TYPE OF RUN
○ LONG, SLOW DISTANCE RUN
○ SPEED/TRACK WORKOUT
○ MY REGULAR RUN

WHERE
○ INDOOR
○ OUTDOOR

ROUTE

DISTANCE

TIME OF DAY/NIGHT

TIME   PACE   WEATHER

EFFORT
| 1 EASY | 2 EASY+ | 3 OK! | 4 OOF | 5 OMG |

COMMENTS

FRIDAY

STRETCHING/WARM-UP

GOAL(S) FOR WORKOUT

TYPE OF RUN
○ LONG, SLOW DISTANCE RUN
○ SPEED/TRACK WORKOUT
○ MY REGULAR RUN

WHERE
○ INDOOR
○ OUTDOOR

ROUTE

DISTANCE

TIME OF DAY/NIGHT

TIME   PACE   WEATHER

EFFORT
| 1 EASY | 2 EASY+ | 3 OK! | 4 OOF | 5 OMG |

COMMENTS

SATURDAY

STRETCHING/WARM-UP

GOAL(S) FOR WORKOUT

TYPE OF RUN
○ LONG, SLOW DISTANCE RUN
○ SPEED/TRACK WORKOUT
○ MY REGULAR RUN

WHERE
○ INDOOR
○ OUTDOOR

ROUTE

DISTANCE

TIME OF DAY/NIGHT

TIME   PACE   WEATHER

EFFORT
| 1 EASY | 2 EASY+ | 3 OK! | 4 OOF | 5 OMG |

COMMENTS

SUNDAY

STRETCHING/WARM-UP

GOAL(S) FOR WORKOUT

TYPE OF RUN
○ LONG, SLOW DISTANCE RUN
○ SPEED/TRACK WORKOUT
○ MY REGULAR RUN

WHERE
○ INDOOR
○ OUTDOOR

ROUTE

DISTANCE

TIME OF DAY/NIGHT

TIME   PACE   WEATHER

EFFORT
| 1 EASY | 2 EASY+ | 3 OK! | 4 OOF | 5 OMG |

COMMENTS

WEEK 26

BEGIN DATE

END DATE

TOTAL MILEAGE THIS WEEK

MONDAY

STRETCHING/WARM-UP

GOAL(S) FOR WORKOUT

TYPE OF RUN
- ○ LONG, SLOW DISTANCE RUN
- ○ SPEED/TRACK WORKOUT
- ○ MY REGULAR RUN

WHERE
- ○ INDOOR
- ○ OUTDOOR

ROUTE

DISTANCE

TIME OF DAY/NIGHT

TIME   PACE   WEATHER

EFFORT

| 1 EASY | 2 EASY+ | 3 OK! | 4 OOF | 5 OMG |

COMMENTS

TUESDAY

STRETCHING/WARM-UP

GOAL(S) FOR WORKOUT

TYPE OF RUN
- ○ LONG, SLOW DISTANCE RUN
- ○ SPEED/TRACK WORKOUT
- ○ MY REGULAR RUN

WHERE
- ○ INDOOR
- ○ OUTDOOR

ROUTE

DISTANCE

TIME OF DAY/NIGHT

TIME   PACE   WEATHER

EFFORT

| 1 EASY | 2 EASY+ | 3 OK! | 4 OOF | 5 OMG |

COMMENTS

WEDNESDAY

STRETCHING/WARM-UP

GOAL(S) FOR WORKOUT

TYPE OF RUN
- ○ LONG, SLOW DISTANCE RUN
- ○ SPEED/TRACK WORKOUT
- ○ MY REGULAR RUN

WHERE
- ○ INDOOR
- ○ OUTDOOR

ROUTE

DISTANCE

TIME OF DAY/NIGHT

TIME   PACE   WEATHER

EFFORT

| 1 EASY | 2 EASY+ | 3 OK! | 4 OOF | 5 OMG |

COMMENTS

THURSDAY

STRETCHING/WARM-UP

GOAL(S) FOR WORKOUT

TYPE OF RUN
- ○ LONG, SLOW DISTANCE RUN
- ○ SPEED/TRACK WORKOUT
- ○ MY REGULAR RUN

WHERE
- ○ INDOOR
- ○ OUTDOOR

ROUTE

DISTANCE

TIME OF DAY/NIGHT

TIME   PACE   WEATHER

EFFORT
| 1 EASY | 2 EASY+ | 3 OK! | 4 OOF | 5 OMG |

COMMENTS

FRIDAY

STRETCHING/WARM-UP

GOAL(S) FOR WORKOUT

TYPE OF RUN
- ○ LONG, SLOW DISTANCE RUN
- ○ SPEED/TRACK WORKOUT
- ○ MY REGULAR RUN

WHERE
- ○ INDOOR
- ○ OUTDOOR

ROUTE

DISTANCE

TIME OF DAY/NIGHT

TIME   PACE   WEATHER

EFFORT
| 1 EASY | 2 EASY+ | 3 OK! | 4 OOF | 5 OMG |

COMMENTS

SATURDAY

STRETCHING/WARM-UP

GOAL(S) FOR WORKOUT

TYPE OF RUN
- ○ LONG, SLOW DISTANCE RUN
- ○ SPEED/TRACK WORKOUT
- ○ MY REGULAR RUN

WHERE
- ○ INDOOR
- ○ OUTDOOR

ROUTE

DISTANCE

TIME OF DAY/NIGHT

TIME   PACE   WEATHER

EFFORT
| 1 EASY | 2 EASY+ | 3 OK! | 4 OOF | 5 OMG |

COMMENTS

SUNDAY

STRETCHING/WARM-UP

GOAL(S) FOR WORKOUT

TYPE OF RUN
- ○ LONG, SLOW DISTANCE RUN
- ○ SPEED/TRACK WORKOUT
- ○ MY REGULAR RUN

WHERE
- ○ INDOOR
- ○ OUTDOOR

ROUTE

DISTANCE

TIME OF DAY/NIGHT

TIME   PACE   WEATHER

EFFORT
| 1 EASY | 2 EASY+ | 3 OK! | 4 OOF | 5 OMG |

COMMENTS

WEEK 27

BEGIN DATE

END DATE

TOTAL MILEAGE THIS WEEK

MONDAY

STRETCHING/WARM-UP

GOAL(S) FOR WORKOUT

TYPE OF RUN
- ○ LONG, SLOW DISTANCE RUN
- ○ SPEED/TRACK WORKOUT
- ○ MY REGULAR RUN

WHERE
- ○ INDOOR
- ○ OUTDOOR

ROUTE

DISTANCE

TIME OF DAY/NIGHT

TIME

PACE

WEATHER

EFFORT

| 1 EASY | 2 EASY+ | 3 OK! | 4 OOF | 5 OMG |

COMMENTS

TUESDAY

STRETCHING/WARM-UP

GOAL(S) FOR WORKOUT

TYPE OF RUN
- ○ LONG, SLOW DISTANCE RUN
- ○ SPEED/TRACK WORKOUT
- ○ MY REGULAR RUN

WHERE
- ○ INDOOR
- ○ OUTDOOR

ROUTE

DISTANCE

TIME OF DAY/NIGHT

TIME

PACE

WEATHER

EFFORT

| 1 EASY | 2 EASY+ | 3 OK! | 4 OOF | 5 OMG |

COMMENTS

WEDNESDAY

STRETCHING/WARM-UP

GOAL(S) FOR WORKOUT

TYPE OF RUN
- ○ LONG, SLOW DISTANCE RUN
- ○ SPEED/TRACK WORKOUT
- ○ MY REGULAR RUN

WHERE
- ○ INDOOR
- ○ OUTDOOR

ROUTE

DISTANCE

TIME OF DAY/NIGHT

TIME

PACE

WEATHER

EFFORT

| 1 EASY | 2 EASY+ | 3 OK! | 4 OOF | 5 OMG |

COMMENTS

THURSDAY

STRETCHING/WARM-UP

DISTANCE

TIME OF DAY/NIGHT

GOAL(S) FOR WORKOUT

TIME　　　**PACE**　　　**WEATHER**

TYPE OF RUN
- ○ LONG, SLOW DISTANCE RUN
- ○ SPEED/TRACK WORKOUT
- ○ MY REGULAR RUN

WHERE
- ○ INDOOR
- ○ OUTDOOR

EFFORT
| 1 EASY | 2 EASY+ | 3 OK! | 4 OOF | 5 OMG |

COMMENTS

ROUTE

FRIDAY

STRETCHING/WARM-UP

DISTANCE

TIME OF DAY/NIGHT

GOAL(S) FOR WORKOUT

TIME　　　**PACE**　　　**WEATHER**

TYPE OF RUN
- ○ LONG, SLOW DISTANCE RUN
- ○ SPEED/TRACK WORKOUT
- ○ MY REGULAR RUN

WHERE
- ○ INDOOR
- ○ OUTDOOR

EFFORT
| 1 EASY | 2 EASY+ | 3 OK! | 4 OOF | 5 OMG |

COMMENTS

ROUTE

SATURDAY

STRETCHING/WARM-UP

DISTANCE

TIME OF DAY/NIGHT

GOAL(S) FOR WORKOUT

TIME　　　**PACE**　　　**WEATHER**

TYPE OF RUN
- ○ LONG, SLOW DISTANCE RUN
- ○ SPEED/TRACK WORKOUT
- ○ MY REGULAR RUN

WHERE
- ○ INDOOR
- ○ OUTDOOR

EFFORT
| 1 EASY | 2 EASY+ | 3 OK! | 4 OOF | 5 OMG |

COMMENTS

ROUTE

SUNDAY

STRETCHING/WARM-UP

DISTANCE

TIME OF DAY/NIGHT

GOAL(S) FOR WORKOUT

TIME　　　**PACE**　　　**WEATHER**

TYPE OF RUN
- ○ LONG, SLOW DISTANCE RUN
- ○ SPEED/TRACK WORKOUT
- ○ MY REGULAR RUN

WHERE
- ○ INDOOR
- ○ OUTDOOR

EFFORT
| 1 EASY | 2 EASY+ | 3 OK! | 4 OOF | 5 OMG |

COMMENTS

ROUTE

WEEK 28

BEGIN DATE

END DATE

TOTAL MILEAGE THIS WEEK

MONDAY

STRETCHING/WARM-UP

GOAL(S) FOR WORKOUT

TYPE OF RUN
- ○ LONG, SLOW DISTANCE RUN
- ○ SPEED/TRACK WORKOUT
- ○ MY REGULAR RUN

WHERE
- ○ INDOOR
- ○ OUTDOOR

ROUTE

DISTANCE

TIME OF DAY/NIGHT

TIME

PACE

WEATHER

EFFORT

| 1 EASY | 2 EASY+ | 3 OK! | 4 OOF | 5 OMG |

COMMENTS

TUESDAY

STRETCHING/WARM-UP

GOAL(S) FOR WORKOUT

TYPE OF RUN
- ○ LONG, SLOW DISTANCE RUN
- ○ SPEED/TRACK WORKOUT
- ○ MY REGULAR RUN

WHERE
- ○ INDOOR
- ○ OUTDOOR

ROUTE

DISTANCE

TIME OF DAY/NIGHT

TIME

PACE

WEATHER

EFFORT

| 1 EASY | 2 EASY+ | 3 OK! | 4 OOF | 5 OMG |

COMMENTS

WEDNESDAY

STRETCHING/WARM-UP

GOAL(S) FOR WORKOUT

TYPE OF RUN
- ○ LONG, SLOW DISTANCE RUN
- ○ SPEED/TRACK WORKOUT
- ○ MY REGULAR RUN

WHERE
- ○ INDOOR
- ○ OUTDOOR

ROUTE

DISTANCE

TIME OF DAY/NIGHT

TIME

PACE

WEATHER

EFFORT

| 1 EASY | 2 EASY+ | 3 OK! | 4 OOF | 5 OMG |

COMMENTS

THURSDAY

STRETCHING/WARM-UP

GOAL(S) FOR WORKOUT

TYPE OF RUN
- ○ LONG, SLOW DISTANCE RUN
- ○ SPEED/TRACK WORKOUT
- ○ MY REGULAR RUN

WHERE
- ○ INDOOR
- ○ OUTDOOR

ROUTE

DISTANCE

TIME OF DAY/NIGHT

TIME   PACE   WEATHER

EFFORT

| 1 EASY | 2 EASY+ | 3 OK! | 4 OOF | 5 OMG |

COMMENTS

FRIDAY

STRETCHING/WARM-UP

GOAL(S) FOR WORKOUT

TYPE OF RUN
- ○ LONG, SLOW DISTANCE RUN
- ○ SPEED/TRACK WORKOUT
- ○ MY REGULAR RUN

WHERE
- ○ INDOOR
- ○ OUTDOOR

ROUTE

DISTANCE

TIME OF DAY/NIGHT

TIME   PACE   WEATHER

EFFORT

| 1 EASY | 2 EASY+ | 3 OK! | 4 OOF | 5 OMG |

COMMENTS

SATURDAY

STRETCHING/WARM-UP

GOAL(S) FOR WORKOUT

TYPE OF RUN
- ○ LONG, SLOW DISTANCE RUN
- ○ SPEED/TRACK WORKOUT
- ○ MY REGULAR RUN

WHERE
- ○ INDOOR
- ○ OUTDOOR

ROUTE

DISTANCE

TIME OF DAY/NIGHT

TIME   PACE   WEATHER

EFFORT

| 1 EASY | 2 EASY+ | 3 OK! | 4 OOF | 5 OMG |

COMMENTS

SUNDAY

STRETCHING/WARM-UP

GOAL(S) FOR WORKOUT

TYPE OF RUN
- ○ LONG, SLOW DISTANCE RUN
- ○ SPEED/TRACK WORKOUT
- ○ MY REGULAR RUN

WHERE
- ○ INDOOR
- ○ OUTDOOR

ROUTE

DISTANCE

TIME OF DAY/NIGHT

TIME   PACE   WEATHER

EFFORT

| 1 EASY | 2 EASY+ | 3 OK! | 4 OOF | 5 OMG |

COMMENTS

WEEK 29

BEGIN DATE

END DATE

TOTAL MILEAGE THIS WEEK

MONDAY

STRETCHING/WARM-UP

GOAL(S) FOR WORKOUT

TYPE OF RUN
- ○ LONG, SLOW DISTANCE RUN
- ○ SPEED/TRACK WORKOUT
- ○ MY REGULAR RUN

WHERE
- ○ INDOOR
- ○ OUTDOOR

ROUTE

DISTANCE

TIME OF DAY/NIGHT

TIME

PACE

WEATHER

EFFORT

| 1 EASY | 2 EASY+ | 3 OK! | 4 OOF | 5 OMG |

COMMENTS

TUESDAY

STRETCHING/WARM-UP

GOAL(S) FOR WORKOUT

TYPE OF RUN
- ○ LONG, SLOW DISTANCE RUN
- ○ SPEED/TRACK WORKOUT
- ○ MY REGULAR RUN

WHERE
- ○ INDOOR
- ○ OUTDOOR

ROUTE

DISTANCE

TIME OF DAY/NIGHT

TIME

PACE

WEATHER

EFFORT

| 1 EASY | 2 EASY+ | 3 OK! | 4 OOF | 5 OMG |

COMMENTS

WEDNESDAY

STRETCHING/WARM-UP

GOAL(S) FOR WORKOUT

TYPE OF RUN
- ○ LONG, SLOW DISTANCE RUN
- ○ SPEED/TRACK WORKOUT
- ○ MY REGULAR RUN

WHERE
- ○ INDOOR
- ○ OUTDOOR

ROUTE

DISTANCE

TIME OF DAY/NIGHT

TIME

PACE

WEATHER

EFFORT

| 1 EASY | 2 EASY+ | 3 OK! | 4 OOF | 5 OMG |

COMMENTS

THURSDAY

STRETCHING/WARM-UP

GOAL(S) FOR WORKOUT

TYPE OF RUN
○ LONG, SLOW DISTANCE RUN
○ SPEED/TRACK WORKOUT
○ MY REGULAR RUN

WHERE
○ INDOOR
○ OUTDOOR

ROUTE

DISTANCE

TIME OF DAY/NIGHT

TIME

PACE

WEATHER

EFFORT

| 1 EASY | 2 EASY+ | 3 OK! | 4 OOF | 5 OMG |

COMMENTS

FRIDAY

STRETCHING/WARM-UP

GOAL(S) FOR WORKOUT

TYPE OF RUN
○ LONG, SLOW DISTANCE RUN
○ SPEED/TRACK WORKOUT
○ MY REGULAR RUN

WHERE
○ INDOOR
○ OUTDOOR

ROUTE

DISTANCE

TIME OF DAY/NIGHT

TIME

PACE

WEATHER

EFFORT

| 1 EASY | 2 EASY+ | 3 OK! | 4 OOF | 5 OMG |

COMMENTS

SATURDAY

STRETCHING/WARM-UP

GOAL(S) FOR WORKOUT

TYPE OF RUN
○ LONG, SLOW DISTANCE RUN
○ SPEED/TRACK WORKOUT
○ MY REGULAR RUN

WHERE
○ INDOOR
○ OUTDOOR

ROUTE

DISTANCE

TIME OF DAY/NIGHT

TIME

PACE

WEATHER

EFFORT

| 1 EASY | 2 EASY+ | 3 OK! | 4 OOF | 5 OMG |

COMMENTS

SUNDAY

STRETCHING/WARM-UP

GOAL(S) FOR WORKOUT

TYPE OF RUN
○ LONG, SLOW DISTANCE RUN
○ SPEED/TRACK WORKOUT
○ MY REGULAR RUN

WHERE
○ INDOOR
○ OUTDOOR

ROUTE

DISTANCE

TIME OF DAY/NIGHT

TIME

PACE

WEATHER

EFFORT

| 1 EASY | 2 EASY+ | 3 OK! | 4 OOF | 5 OMG |

COMMENTS

WEEK 30

BEGIN DATE

END DATE

TOTAL MILEAGE THIS WEEK

MONDAY

STRETCHING/WARM-UP

DISTANCE

TIME OF DAY/NIGHT

GOAL(S) FOR WORKOUT

TIME

PACE

WEATHER

TYPE OF RUN
- ○ LONG, SLOW DISTANCE RUN
- ○ SPEED/TRACK WORKOUT
- ○ MY REGULAR RUN

WHERE
- ○ INDOOR
- ○ OUTDOOR

EFFORT

| 1 EASY | 2 EASY+ | 3 OK! | 4 OOF | 5 OMG |

COMMENTS

ROUTE

TUESDAY

STRETCHING/WARM-UP

DISTANCE

TIME OF DAY/NIGHT

GOAL(S) FOR WORKOUT

TIME

PACE

WEATHER

TYPE OF RUN
- ○ LONG, SLOW DISTANCE RUN
- ○ SPEED/TRACK WORKOUT
- ○ MY REGULAR RUN

WHERE
- ○ INDOOR
- ○ OUTDOOR

EFFORT

| 1 EASY | 2 EASY+ | 3 OK! | 4 OOF | 5 OMG |

COMMENTS

ROUTE

WEDNESDAY

STRETCHING/WARM-UP

DISTANCE

TIME OF DAY/NIGHT

GOAL(S) FOR WORKOUT

TIME

PACE

WEATHER

TYPE OF RUN
- ○ LONG, SLOW DISTANCE RUN
- ○ SPEED/TRACK WORKOUT
- ○ MY REGULAR RUN

WHERE
- ○ INDOOR
- ○ OUTDOOR

EFFORT

| 1 EASY | 2 EASY+ | 3 OK! | 4 OOF | 5 OMG |

COMMENTS

ROUTE

THURSDAY

STRETCHING/WARM-UP

GOAL(S) FOR WORKOUT

TYPE OF RUN
- ○ LONG, SLOW DISTANCE RUN
- ○ SPEED/TRACK WORKOUT
- ○ MY REGULAR RUN

WHERE
- ○ INDOOR
- ○ OUTDOOR

ROUTE

DISTANCE

TIME OF DAY/NIGHT

TIME   PACE   WEATHER

EFFORT

| 1 EASY | 2 EASY+ | 3 OK! | 4 OOF | 5 OMG |

COMMENTS

FRIDAY

STRETCHING/WARM-UP

GOAL(S) FOR WORKOUT

TYPE OF RUN
- ○ LONG, SLOW DISTANCE RUN
- ○ SPEED/TRACK WORKOUT
- ○ MY REGULAR RUN

WHERE
- ○ INDOOR
- ○ OUTDOOR

ROUTE

DISTANCE

TIME OF DAY/NIGHT

TIME   PACE   WEATHER

EFFORT

| 1 EASY | 2 EASY+ | 3 OK! | 4 OOF | 5 OMG |

COMMENTS

SATURDAY

STRETCHING/WARM-UP

GOAL(S) FOR WORKOUT

TYPE OF RUN
- ○ LONG, SLOW DISTANCE RUN
- ○ SPEED/TRACK WORKOUT
- ○ MY REGULAR RUN

WHERE
- ○ INDOOR
- ○ OUTDOOR

ROUTE

DISTANCE

TIME OF DAY/NIGHT

TIME   PACE   WEATHER

EFFORT

| 1 EASY | 2 EASY+ | 3 OK! | 4 OOF | 5 OMG |

COMMENTS

SUNDAY

STRETCHING/WARM-UP

GOAL(S) FOR WORKOUT

TYPE OF RUN
- ○ LONG, SLOW DISTANCE RUN
- ○ SPEED/TRACK WORKOUT
- ○ MY REGULAR RUN

WHERE
- ○ INDOOR
- ○ OUTDOOR

ROUTE

DISTANCE

TIME OF DAY/NIGHT

TIME   PACE   WEATHER

EFFORT

| 1 EASY | 2 EASY+ | 3 OK! | 4 OOF | 5 OMG |

COMMENTS

WEEK 31

BEGIN DATE

END DATE

TOTAL MILEAGE THIS WEEK

MONDAY

STRETCHING/WARM-UP	DISTANCE	TIME OF DAY/NIGHT

GOAL(S) FOR WORKOUT	TIME	PACE	WEATHER

TYPE OF RUN
- ○ LONG, SLOW DISTANCE RUN
- ○ SPEED/TRACK WORKOUT
- ○ MY REGULAR RUN

WHERE
- ○ INDOOR
- ○ OUTDOOR

EFFORT

1 EASY	2 EASY+	3 OK!	4 OOF	5 OMG

COMMENTS

ROUTE

TUESDAY

STRETCHING/WARM-UP	DISTANCE	TIME OF DAY/NIGHT

GOAL(S) FOR WORKOUT	TIME	PACE	WEATHER

TYPE OF RUN
- ○ LONG, SLOW DISTANCE RUN
- ○ SPEED/TRACK WORKOUT
- ○ MY REGULAR RUN

WHERE
- ○ INDOOR
- ○ OUTDOOR

EFFORT

1 EASY	2 EASY+	3 OK!	4 OOF	5 OMG

COMMENTS

ROUTE

WEDNESDAY

STRETCHING/WARM-UP	DISTANCE	TIME OF DAY/NIGHT

GOAL(S) FOR WORKOUT	TIME	PACE	WEATHER

TYPE OF RUN
- ○ LONG, SLOW DISTANCE RUN
- ○ SPEED/TRACK WORKOUT
- ○ MY REGULAR RUN

WHERE
- ○ INDOOR
- ○ OUTDOOR

EFFORT

1 EASY	2 EASY+	3 OK!	4 OOF	5 OMG

COMMENTS

ROUTE

THURSDAY

STRETCHING/WARM-UP

GOAL(S) FOR WORKOUT

TYPE OF RUN
- ○ LONG, SLOW DISTANCE RUN
- ○ SPEED/TRACK WORKOUT
- ○ MY REGULAR RUN

WHERE
- ○ INDOOR
- ○ OUTDOOR

ROUTE

DISTANCE

TIME OF DAY/NIGHT

TIME   PACE   WEATHER

EFFORT
| 1 EASY | 2 EASY+ | 3 OK! | 4 OOF | 5 OMG |

COMMENTS

FRIDAY

STRETCHING/WARM-UP

GOAL(S) FOR WORKOUT

TYPE OF RUN
- ○ LONG, SLOW DISTANCE RUN
- ○ SPEED/TRACK WORKOUT
- ○ MY REGULAR RUN

WHERE
- ○ INDOOR
- ○ OUTDOOR

ROUTE

DISTANCE

TIME OF DAY/NIGHT

TIME   PACE   WEATHER

EFFORT
| 1 EASY | 2 EASY+ | 3 OK! | 4 OOF | 5 OMG |

COMMENTS

SATURDAY

STRETCHING/WARM-UP

GOAL(S) FOR WORKOUT

TYPE OF RUN
- ○ LONG, SLOW DISTANCE RUN
- ○ SPEED/TRACK WORKOUT
- ○ MY REGULAR RUN

WHERE
- ○ INDOOR
- ○ OUTDOOR

ROUTE

DISTANCE

TIME OF DAY/NIGHT

TIME   PACE   WEATHER

EFFORT
| 1 EASY | 2 EASY+ | 3 OK! | 4 OOF | 5 OMG |

COMMENTS

SUNDAY

STRETCHING/WARM-UP

GOAL(S) FOR WORKOUT

TYPE OF RUN
- ○ LONG, SLOW DISTANCE RUN
- ○ SPEED/TRACK WORKOUT
- ○ MY REGULAR RUN

WHERE
- ○ INDOOR
- ○ OUTDOOR

ROUTE

DISTANCE

TIME OF DAY/NIGHT

TIME   PACE   WEATHER

EFFORT
| 1 EASY | 2 EASY+ | 3 OK! | 4 OOF | 5 OMG |

COMMENTS

WEEK 32

BEGIN DATE	END DATE

TOTAL MILEAGE THIS WEEK

MONDAY

STRETCHING/WARM-UP

GOAL(S) FOR WORKOUT

TYPE OF RUN
- ○ LONG, SLOW DISTANCE RUN
- ○ SPEED/TRACK WORKOUT
- ○ MY REGULAR RUN

WHERE
- ○ INDOOR
- ○ OUTDOOR

ROUTE

DISTANCE

TIME OF DAY/NIGHT

TIME   PACE   WEATHER

EFFORT
| 1 EASY | 2 EASY+ | 3 OK! | 4 OOF | 5 OMG |

COMMENTS

TUESDAY

STRETCHING/WARM-UP

GOAL(S) FOR WORKOUT

TYPE OF RUN
- ○ LONG, SLOW DISTANCE RUN
- ○ SPEED/TRACK WORKOUT
- ○ MY REGULAR RUN

WHERE
- ○ INDOOR
- ○ OUTDOOR

ROUTE

DISTANCE

TIME OF DAY/NIGHT

TIME   PACE   WEATHER

EFFORT
| 1 EASY | 2 EASY+ | 3 OK! | 4 OOF | 5 OMG |

COMMENTS

WEDNESDAY

STRETCHING/WARM-UP

GOAL(S) FOR WORKOUT

TYPE OF RUN
- ○ LONG, SLOW DISTANCE RUN
- ○ SPEED/TRACK WORKOUT
- ○ MY REGULAR RUN

WHERE
- ○ INDOOR
- ○ OUTDOOR

ROUTE

DISTANCE

TIME OF DAY/NIGHT

TIME   PACE   WEATHER

EFFORT
| 1 EASY | 2 EASY+ | 3 OK! | 4 OOF | 5 OMG |

COMMENTS

THURSDAY

STRETCHING/WARM-UP

GOAL(S) FOR WORKOUT

TYPE OF RUN
- ○ LONG, SLOW DISTANCE RUN
- ○ SPEED/TRACK WORKOUT
- ○ MY REGULAR RUN

WHERE
- ○ INDOOR
- ○ OUTDOOR

ROUTE

DISTANCE

TIME OF DAY/NIGHT

TIME | PACE | WEATHER

EFFORT

| 1 EASY | 2 EASY+ | 3 OK! | 4 OOF | 5 OMG |

COMMENTS

FRIDAY

STRETCHING/WARM-UP

GOAL(S) FOR WORKOUT

TYPE OF RUN
- ○ LONG, SLOW DISTANCE RUN
- ○ SPEED/TRACK WORKOUT
- ○ MY REGULAR RUN

WHERE
- ○ INDOOR
- ○ OUTDOOR

ROUTE

DISTANCE

TIME OF DAY/NIGHT

TIME | PACE | WEATHER

EFFORT

| 1 EASY | 2 EASY+ | 3 OK! | 4 OOF | 5 OMG |

COMMENTS

SATURDAY

STRETCHING/WARM-UP

GOAL(S) FOR WORKOUT

TYPE OF RUN
- ○ LONG, SLOW DISTANCE RUN
- ○ SPEED/TRACK WORKOUT
- ○ MY REGULAR RUN

WHERE
- ○ INDOOR
- ○ OUTDOOR

ROUTE

DISTANCE

TIME OF DAY/NIGHT

TIME | PACE | WEATHER

EFFORT

| 1 EASY | 2 EASY+ | 3 OK! | 4 OOF | 5 OMG |

COMMENTS

SUNDAY

STRETCHING/WARM-UP

GOAL(S) FOR WORKOUT

TYPE OF RUN
- ○ LONG, SLOW DISTANCE RUN
- ○ SPEED/TRACK WORKOUT
- ○ MY REGULAR RUN

WHERE
- ○ INDOOR
- ○ OUTDOOR

ROUTE

DISTANCE

TIME OF DAY/NIGHT

TIME | PACE | WEATHER

EFFORT

| 1 EASY | 2 EASY+ | 3 OK! | 4 OOF | 5 OMG |

COMMENTS

WEEK 33

BEGIN DATE

END DATE

TOTAL MILEAGE THIS WEEK

MONDAY

STRETCHING/WARM-UP

GOAL(S) FOR WORKOUT

TYPE OF RUN
- ○ LONG, SLOW DISTANCE RUN
- ○ SPEED/TRACK WORKOUT
- ○ MY REGULAR RUN

WHERE
- ○ INDOOR
- ○ OUTDOOR

ROUTE

DISTANCE

TIME OF DAY/NIGHT

TIME   PACE   WEATHER

EFFORT

| 1 EASY | 2 EASY+ | 3 OK! | 4 OOF | 5 OMG |

COMMENTS

TUESDAY

STRETCHING/WARM-UP

GOAL(S) FOR WORKOUT

TYPE OF RUN
- ○ LONG, SLOW DISTANCE RUN
- ○ SPEED/TRACK WORKOUT
- ○ MY REGULAR RUN

WHERE
- ○ INDOOR
- ○ OUTDOOR

ROUTE

DISTANCE

TIME OF DAY/NIGHT

TIME   PACE   WEATHER

EFFORT

| 1 EASY | 2 EASY+ | 3 OK! | 4 OOF | 5 OMG |

COMMENTS

WEDNESDAY

STRETCHING/WARM-UP

GOAL(S) FOR WORKOUT

TYPE OF RUN
- ○ LONG, SLOW DISTANCE RUN
- ○ SPEED/TRACK WORKOUT
- ○ MY REGULAR RUN

WHERE
- ○ INDOOR
- ○ OUTDOOR

ROUTE

DISTANCE

TIME OF DAY/NIGHT

TIME   PACE   WEATHER

EFFORT

| 1 EASY | 2 EASY+ | 3 OK! | 4 OOF | 5 OMG |

COMMENTS

THURSDAY

STRETCHING/WARM-UP

GOAL(S) FOR WORKOUT

TYPE OF RUN
- ○ LONG, SLOW DISTANCE RUN
- ○ SPEED/TRACK WORKOUT
- ○ MY REGULAR RUN

WHERE
- ○ INDOOR
- ○ OUTDOOR

ROUTE

DISTANCE

TIME OF DAY/NIGHT

TIME

PACE

WEATHER

EFFORT

1 EASY	2 EASY+	3 OK!	4 OOF	5 OMG

COMMENTS

FRIDAY

STRETCHING/WARM-UP

GOAL(S) FOR WORKOUT

TYPE OF RUN
- ○ LONG, SLOW DISTANCE RUN
- ○ SPEED/TRACK WORKOUT
- ○ MY REGULAR RUN

WHERE
- ○ INDOOR
- ○ OUTDOOR

ROUTE

DISTANCE

TIME OF DAY/NIGHT

TIME

PACE

WEATHER

EFFORT

1 EASY	2 EASY+	3 OK!	4 OOF	5 OMG

COMMENTS

SATURDAY

STRETCHING/WARM-UP

GOAL(S) FOR WORKOUT

TYPE OF RUN
- ○ LONG, SLOW DISTANCE RUN
- ○ SPEED/TRACK WORKOUT
- ○ MY REGULAR RUN

WHERE
- ○ INDOOR
- ○ OUTDOOR

ROUTE

DISTANCE

TIME OF DAY/NIGHT

TIME

PACE

WEATHER

EFFORT

1 EASY	2 EASY+	3 OK!	4 OOF	5 OMG

COMMENTS

SUNDAY

STRETCHING/WARM-UP

GOAL(S) FOR WORKOUT

TYPE OF RUN
- ○ LONG, SLOW DISTANCE RUN
- ○ SPEED/TRACK WORKOUT
- ○ MY REGULAR RUN

WHERE
- ○ INDOOR
- ○ OUTDOOR

ROUTE

DISTANCE

TIME OF DAY/NIGHT

TIME

PACE

WEATHER

EFFORT

1 EASY	2 EASY+	3 OK!	4 OOF	5 OMG

COMMENTS

WEEK 34

BEGIN DATE	END DATE

TOTAL MILEAGE THIS WEEK

MONDAY

STRETCHING/WARM-UP

GOAL(S) FOR WORKOUT

TYPE OF RUN
- ○ LONG, SLOW DISTANCE RUN
- ○ SPEED/TRACK WORKOUT
- ○ MY REGULAR RUN

WHERE
- ○ INDOOR
- ○ OUTDOOR

ROUTE

DISTANCE

TIME OF DAY/NIGHT

TIME   PACE   WEATHER

EFFORT

1 EASY	2 EASY+	3 OK!	4 OOF	5 OMG

COMMENTS

TUESDAY

STRETCHING/WARM-UP

GOAL(S) FOR WORKOUT

TYPE OF RUN
- ○ LONG, SLOW DISTANCE RUN
- ○ SPEED/TRACK WORKOUT
- ○ MY REGULAR RUN

WHERE
- ○ INDOOR
- ○ OUTDOOR

ROUTE

DISTANCE

TIME OF DAY/NIGHT

TIME   PACE   WEATHER

EFFORT

1 EASY	2 EASY+	3 OK!	4 OOF	5 OMG

COMMENTS

WEDNESDAY

STRETCHING/WARM-UP

GOAL(S) FOR WORKOUT

TYPE OF RUN
- ○ LONG, SLOW DISTANCE RUN
- ○ SPEED/TRACK WORKOUT
- ○ MY REGULAR RUN

WHERE
- ○ INDOOR
- ○ OUTDOOR

ROUTE

DISTANCE

TIME OF DAY/NIGHT

TIME   PACE   WEATHER

EFFORT

1 EASY	2 EASY+	3 OK!	4 OOF	5 OMG

COMMENTS

THURSDAY

STRETCHING/WARM-UP

GOAL(S) FOR WORKOUT

TYPE OF RUN
- ○ LONG, SLOW DISTANCE RUN
- ○ SPEED/TRACK WORKOUT
- ○ MY REGULAR RUN

WHERE
- ○ INDOOR
- ○ OUTDOOR

ROUTE

DISTANCE

TIME OF DAY/NIGHT

TIME   **PACE**   **WEATHER**

EFFORT

| 1 EASY | 2 EASY+ | 3 OK! | 4 OOF | 5 OMG |

COMMENTS

FRIDAY

STRETCHING/WARM-UP

GOAL(S) FOR WORKOUT

TYPE OF RUN
- ○ LONG, SLOW DISTANCE RUN
- ○ SPEED/TRACK WORKOUT
- ○ MY REGULAR RUN

WHERE
- ○ INDOOR
- ○ OUTDOOR

ROUTE

DISTANCE

TIME OF DAY/NIGHT

TIME   **PACE**   **WEATHER**

EFFORT

| 1 EASY | 2 EASY+ | 3 OK! | 4 OOF | 5 OMG |

COMMENTS

SATURDAY

STRETCHING/WARM-UP

GOAL(S) FOR WORKOUT

TYPE OF RUN
- ○ LONG, SLOW DISTANCE RUN
- ○ SPEED/TRACK WORKOUT
- ○ MY REGULAR RUN

WHERE
- ○ INDOOR
- ○ OUTDOOR

ROUTE

DISTANCE

TIME OF DAY/NIGHT

TIME   **PACE**   **WEATHER**

EFFORT

| 1 EASY | 2 EASY+ | 3 OK! | 4 OOF | 5 OMG |

COMMENTS

SUNDAY

STRETCHING/WARM-UP

GOAL(S) FOR WORKOUT

TYPE OF RUN
- ○ LONG, SLOW DISTANCE RUN
- ○ SPEED/TRACK WORKOUT
- ○ MY REGULAR RUN

WHERE
- ○ INDOOR
- ○ OUTDOOR

ROUTE

DISTANCE

TIME OF DAY/NIGHT

TIME   **PACE**   **WEATHER**

EFFORT

| 1 EASY | 2 EASY+ | 3 OK! | 4 OOF | 5 OMG |

COMMENTS

BEGIN DATE

END DATE

TOTAL MILEAGE THIS WEEK

MONDAY

STRETCHING/WARM-UP

GOAL(S) FOR WORKOUT

TYPE OF RUN
- LONG, SLOW DISTANCE RUN
- SPEED/TRACK WORKOUT
- MY REGULAR RUN

WHERE
- INDOOR
- OUTDOOR

ROUTE

DISTANCE

TIME OF DAY/NIGHT

TIME   PACE   WEATHER

EFFORT | 1 EASY | 2 EASY+ | 3 OK! | 4 OOF | 5 OMG |

COMMENTS

TUESDAY

STRETCHING/WARM-UP

GOAL(S) FOR WORKOUT

TYPE OF RUN
- LONG, SLOW DISTANCE RUN
- SPEED/TRACK WORKOUT
- MY REGULAR RUN

WHERE
- INDOOR
- OUTDOOR

ROUTE

DISTANCE

TIME OF DAY/NIGHT

TIME   PACE   WEATHER

EFFORT | 1 EASY | 2 EASY+ | 3 OK! | 4 OOF | 5 OMG |

COMMENTS

WEDNESDAY

STRETCHING/WARM-UP

GOAL(S) FOR WORKOUT

TYPE OF RUN
- LONG, SLOW DISTANCE RUN
- SPEED/TRACK WORKOUT
- MY REGULAR RUN

WHERE
- INDOOR
- OUTDOOR

ROUTE

DISTANCE

TIME OF DAY/NIGHT

TIME   PACE   WEATHER

EFFORT | 1 EASY | 2 EASY+ | 3 OK! | 4 OOF | 5 OMG |

COMMENTS

THURSDAY

STRETCHING/WARM-UP

GOAL(S) FOR WORKOUT

TYPE OF RUN
○ LONG, SLOW DISTANCE RUN
○ SPEED/TRACK WORKOUT
○ MY REGULAR RUN

WHERE
○ INDOOR
○ OUTDOOR

ROUTE

DISTANCE

TIME OF DAY/NIGHT

TIME   PACE   WEATHER

EFFORT

| 1 EASY | 2 EASY+ | 3 OK! | 4 OOF | 5 OMG |

COMMENTS

FRIDAY

STRETCHING/WARM-UP

GOAL(S) FOR WORKOUT

TYPE OF RUN
○ LONG, SLOW DISTANCE RUN
○ SPEED/TRACK WORKOUT
○ MY REGULAR RUN

WHERE
○ INDOOR
○ OUTDOOR

ROUTE

DISTANCE

TIME OF DAY/NIGHT

TIME   PACE   WEATHER

EFFORT

| 1 EASY | 2 EASY+ | 3 OK! | 4 OOF | 5 OMG |

COMMENTS

SATURDAY

STRETCHING/WARM-UP

GOAL(S) FOR WORKOUT

TYPE OF RUN
○ LONG, SLOW DISTANCE RUN
○ SPEED/TRACK WORKOUT
○ MY REGULAR RUN

WHERE
○ INDOOR
○ OUTDOOR

ROUTE

DISTANCE

TIME OF DAY/NIGHT

TIME   PACE   WEATHER

EFFORT

| 1 EASY | 2 EASY+ | 3 OK! | 4 OOF | 5 OMG |

COMMENTS

SUNDAY

STRETCHING/WARM-UP

GOAL(S) FOR WORKOUT

TYPE OF RUN
○ LONG, SLOW DISTANCE RUN
○ SPEED/TRACK WORKOUT
○ MY REGULAR RUN

WHERE
○ INDOOR
○ OUTDOOR

ROUTE

DISTANCE

TIME OF DAY/NIGHT

TIME   PACE   WEATHER

EFFORT

| 1 EASY | 2 EASY+ | 3 OK! | 4 OOF | 5 OMG |

COMMENTS

WEEK 36

BEGIN DATE

END DATE

TOTAL MILEAGE THIS WEEK

MONDAY

STRETCHING/WARM-UP

DISTANCE

TIME OF DAY/NIGHT

GOAL(S) FOR WORKOUT

TIME

PACE

WEATHER

TYPE OF RUN
- LONG, SLOW DISTANCE RUN
- SPEED/TRACK WORKOUT
- MY REGULAR RUN

WHERE
- INDOOR
- OUTDOOR

EFFORT

| 1 EASY | 2 EASY+ | 3 OK! | 4 OOF | 5 OMG |

COMMENTS

ROUTE

TUESDAY

STRETCHING/WARM-UP

DISTANCE

TIME OF DAY/NIGHT

GOAL(S) FOR WORKOUT

TIME

PACE

WEATHER

TYPE OF RUN
- LONG, SLOW DISTANCE RUN
- SPEED/TRACK WORKOUT
- MY REGULAR RUN

WHERE
- INDOOR
- OUTDOOR

EFFORT

| 1 EASY | 2 EASY+ | 3 OK! | 4 OOF | 5 OMG |

COMMENTS

ROUTE

WEDNESDAY

STRETCHING/WARM-UP

DISTANCE

TIME OF DAY/NIGHT

GOAL(S) FOR WORKOUT

TIME

PACE

WEATHER

TYPE OF RUN
- LONG, SLOW DISTANCE RUN
- SPEED/TRACK WORKOUT
- MY REGULAR RUN

WHERE
- INDOOR
- OUTDOOR

EFFORT

| 1 EASY | 2 EASY+ | 3 OK! | 4 OOF | 5 OMG |

COMMENTS

ROUTE

THURSDAY

STRETCHING/WARM-UP

GOAL(S) FOR WORKOUT

TYPE OF RUN
○ LONG, SLOW DISTANCE RUN
○ SPEED/TRACK WORKOUT
○ MY REGULAR RUN

WHERE
○ INDOOR
○ OUTDOOR

ROUTE

DISTANCE

TIME OF DAY/NIGHT

TIME　　　**PACE**　　　**WEATHER**

EFFORT
| 1 EASY | 2 EASY+ | 3 OK! | 4 OOF | 5 OMG |

COMMENTS

FRIDAY

STRETCHING/WARM-UP

GOAL(S) FOR WORKOUT

TYPE OF RUN
○ LONG, SLOW DISTANCE RUN
○ SPEED/TRACK WORKOUT
○ MY REGULAR RUN

WHERE
○ INDOOR
○ OUTDOOR

ROUTE

DISTANCE

TIME OF DAY/NIGHT

TIME　　　**PACE**　　　**WEATHER**

EFFORT
| 1 EASY | 2 EASY+ | 3 OK! | 4 OOF | 5 OMG |

COMMENTS

SATURDAY

STRETCHING/WARM-UP

GOAL(S) FOR WORKOUT

TYPE OF RUN
○ LONG, SLOW DISTANCE RUN
○ SPEED/TRACK WORKOUT
○ MY REGULAR RUN

WHERE
○ INDOOR
○ OUTDOOR

ROUTE

DISTANCE

TIME OF DAY/NIGHT

TIME　　　**PACE**　　　**WEATHER**

EFFORT
| 1 EASY | 2 EASY+ | 3 OK! | 4 OOF | 5 OMG |

COMMENTS

SUNDAY

STRETCHING/WARM-UP

GOAL(S) FOR WORKOUT

TYPE OF RUN
○ LONG, SLOW DISTANCE RUN
○ SPEED/TRACK WORKOUT
○ MY REGULAR RUN

WHERE
○ INDOOR
○ OUTDOOR

ROUTE

DISTANCE

TIME OF DAY/NIGHT

TIME　　　**PACE**　　　**WEATHER**

EFFORT
| 1 EASY | 2 EASY+ | 3 OK! | 4 OOF | 5 OMG |

COMMENTS

WEEK 37

BEGIN DATE	END DATE

TOTAL MILEAGE THIS WEEK

MONDAY

STRETCHING/WARM-UP

GOAL(S) FOR WORKOUT

TYPE OF RUN
- ○ LONG, SLOW DISTANCE RUN
- ○ SPEED/TRACK WORKOUT
- ○ MY REGULAR RUN

WHERE
- ○ INDOOR
- ○ OUTDOOR

ROUTE

DISTANCE

TIME OF DAY/NIGHT

TIME   PACE   WEATHER

EFFORT

1 EASY	2 EASY+	3 OK!	4 OOF	5 OMG

COMMENTS

TUESDAY

STRETCHING/WARM-UP

GOAL(S) FOR WORKOUT

TYPE OF RUN
- ○ LONG, SLOW DISTANCE RUN
- ○ SPEED/TRACK WORKOUT
- ○ MY REGULAR RUN

WHERE
- ○ INDOOR
- ○ OUTDOOR

ROUTE

DISTANCE

TIME OF DAY/NIGHT

TIME   PACE   WEATHER

EFFORT

1 EASY	2 EASY+	3 OK!	4 OOF	5 OMG

COMMENTS

WEDNESDAY

STRETCHING/WARM-UP

GOAL(S) FOR WORKOUT

TYPE OF RUN
- ○ LONG, SLOW DISTANCE RUN
- ○ SPEED/TRACK WORKOUT
- ○ MY REGULAR RUN

WHERE
- ○ INDOOR
- ○ OUTDOOR

ROUTE

DISTANCE

TIME OF DAY/NIGHT

TIME   PACE   WEATHER

EFFORT

1 EASY	2 EASY+	3 OK!	4 OOF	5 OMG

COMMENTS

THURSDAY

STRETCHING/WARM-UP

GOAL(S) FOR WORKOUT

TYPE OF RUN
- ○ LONG, SLOW DISTANCE RUN
- ○ SPEED/TRACK WORKOUT
- ○ MY REGULAR RUN

WHERE
- ○ INDOOR
- ○ OUTDOOR

ROUTE

DISTANCE

TIME OF DAY/NIGHT

TIME

PACE

WEATHER

EFFORT

| 1 EASY | 2 EASY+ | 3 OK! | 4 OOF | 5 OMG |

COMMENTS

FRIDAY

STRETCHING/WARM-UP

GOAL(S) FOR WORKOUT

TYPE OF RUN
- ○ LONG, SLOW DISTANCE RUN
- ○ SPEED/TRACK WORKOUT
- ○ MY REGULAR RUN

WHERE
- ○ INDOOR
- ○ OUTDOOR

ROUTE

DISTANCE

TIME OF DAY/NIGHT

TIME

PACE

WEATHER

EFFORT

| 1 EASY | 2 EASY+ | 3 OK! | 4 OOF | 5 OMG |

COMMENTS

SATURDAY

STRETCHING/WARM-UP

GOAL(S) FOR WORKOUT

TYPE OF RUN
- ○ LONG, SLOW DISTANCE RUN
- ○ SPEED/TRACK WORKOUT
- ○ MY REGULAR RUN

WHERE
- ○ INDOOR
- ○ OUTDOOR

ROUTE

DISTANCE

TIME OF DAY/NIGHT

TIME

PACE

WEATHER

EFFORT

| 1 EASY | 2 EASY+ | 3 OK! | 4 OOF | 5 OMG |

COMMENTS

SUNDAY

STRETCHING/WARM-UP

GOAL(S) FOR WORKOUT

TYPE OF RUN
- ○ LONG, SLOW DISTANCE RUN
- ○ SPEED/TRACK WORKOUT
- ○ MY REGULAR RUN

WHERE
- ○ INDOOR
- ○ OUTDOOR

ROUTE

DISTANCE

TIME OF DAY/NIGHT

TIME

PACE

WEATHER

EFFORT

| 1 EASY | 2 EASY+ | 3 OK! | 4 OOF | 5 OMG |

COMMENTS

BEGIN DATE

END DATE

TOTAL MILEAGE THIS WEEK

MONDAY

STRETCHING/WARM-UP

GOAL(S) FOR WORKOUT

TYPE OF RUN
- ○ LONG, SLOW DISTANCE RUN
- ○ SPEED/TRACK WORKOUT
- ○ MY REGULAR RUN

WHERE
- ○ INDOOR
- ○ OUTDOOR

ROUTE

DISTANCE

TIME OF DAY/NIGHT

TIME   PACE   WEATHER

EFFORT

| 1 EASY | 2 EASY+ | 3 OK! | 4 OOF | 5 OMG |

COMMENTS

TUESDAY

STRETCHING/WARM-UP

GOAL(S) FOR WORKOUT

TYPE OF RUN
- ○ LONG, SLOW DISTANCE RUN
- ○ SPEED/TRACK WORKOUT
- ○ MY REGULAR RUN

WHERE
- ○ INDOOR
- ○ OUTDOOR

ROUTE

DISTANCE

TIME OF DAY/NIGHT

TIME   PACE   WEATHER

EFFORT

| 1 EASY | 2 EASY+ | 3 OK! | 4 OOF | 5 OMG |

COMMENTS

WEDNESDAY

STRETCHING/WARM-UP

GOAL(S) FOR WORKOUT

TYPE OF RUN
- ○ LONG, SLOW DISTANCE RUN
- ○ SPEED/TRACK WORKOUT
- ○ MY REGULAR RUN

WHERE
- ○ INDOOR
- ○ OUTDOOR

ROUTE

DISTANCE

TIME OF DAY/NIGHT

TIME   PACE   WEATHER

EFFORT

| 1 EASY | 2 EASY+ | 3 OK! | 4 OOF | 5 OMG |

COMMENTS

THURSDAY

STRETCHING/WARM-UP

GOAL(S) FOR WORKOUT

TYPE OF RUN
- ○ LONG, SLOW DISTANCE RUN
- ○ SPEED/TRACK WORKOUT
- ○ MY REGULAR RUN

WHERE
- ○ INDOOR
- ○ OUTDOOR

ROUTE

DISTANCE

TIME OF DAY/NIGHT

TIME

PACE

WEATHER

EFFORT

| 1 EASY | 2 EASY+ | 3 OK! | 4 OOF | 5 OMG |

COMMENTS

FRIDAY

STRETCHING/WARM-UP

GOAL(S) FOR WORKOUT

TYPE OF RUN
- ○ LONG, SLOW DISTANCE RUN
- ○ SPEED/TRACK WORKOUT
- ○ MY REGULAR RUN

WHERE
- ○ INDOOR
- ○ OUTDOOR

ROUTE

DISTANCE

TIME OF DAY/NIGHT

TIME

PACE

WEATHER

EFFORT

| 1 EASY | 2 EASY+ | 3 OK! | 4 OOF | 5 OMG |

COMMENTS

SATURDAY

STRETCHING/WARM-UP

GOAL(S) FOR WORKOUT

TYPE OF RUN
- ○ LONG, SLOW DISTANCE RUN
- ○ SPEED/TRACK WORKOUT
- ○ MY REGULAR RUN

WHERE
- ○ INDOOR
- ○ OUTDOOR

ROUTE

DISTANCE

TIME OF DAY/NIGHT

TIME

PACE

WEATHER

EFFORT

| 1 EASY | 2 EASY+ | 3 OK! | 4 OOF | 5 OMG |

COMMENTS

SUNDAY

STRETCHING/WARM-UP

GOAL(S) FOR WORKOUT

TYPE OF RUN
- ○ LONG, SLOW DISTANCE RUN
- ○ SPEED/TRACK WORKOUT
- ○ MY REGULAR RUN

WHERE
- ○ INDOOR
- ○ OUTDOOR

ROUTE

DISTANCE

TIME OF DAY/NIGHT

TIME

PACE

WEATHER

EFFORT

| 1 EASY | 2 EASY+ | 3 OK! | 4 OOF | 5 OMG |

COMMENTS

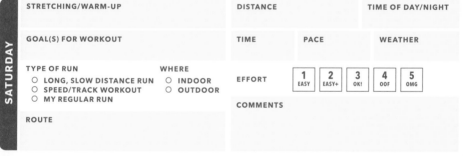

WEEK 39

BEGIN DATE

END DATE

TOTAL MILEAGE THIS WEEK

MONDAY

STRETCHING/WARM-UP

GOAL(S) FOR WORKOUT

TYPE OF RUN
- ○ LONG, SLOW DISTANCE RUN
- ○ SPEED/TRACK WORKOUT
- ○ MY REGULAR RUN

WHERE
- ○ INDOOR
- ○ OUTDOOR

ROUTE

DISTANCE

TIME OF DAY/NIGHT

TIME

PACE

WEATHER

EFFORT

| 1 EASY | 2 EASY+ | 3 OK! | 4 OOF | 5 OMG |

COMMENTS

TUESDAY

STRETCHING/WARM-UP

GOAL(S) FOR WORKOUT

TYPE OF RUN
- ○ LONG, SLOW DISTANCE RUN
- ○ SPEED/TRACK WORKOUT
- ○ MY REGULAR RUN

WHERE
- ○ INDOOR
- ○ OUTDOOR

ROUTE

DISTANCE

TIME OF DAY/NIGHT

TIME

PACE

WEATHER

EFFORT

| 1 EASY | 2 EASY+ | 3 OK! | 4 OOF | 5 OMG |

COMMENTS

WEDNESDAY

STRETCHING/WARM-UP

GOAL(S) FOR WORKOUT

TYPE OF RUN
- ○ LONG, SLOW DISTANCE RUN
- ○ SPEED/TRACK WORKOUT
- ○ MY REGULAR RUN

WHERE
- ○ INDOOR
- ○ OUTDOOR

ROUTE

DISTANCE

TIME OF DAY/NIGHT

TIME

PACE

WEATHER

EFFORT

| 1 EASY | 2 EASY+ | 3 OK! | 4 OOF | 5 OMG |

COMMENTS

THURSDAY

STRETCHING/WARM-UP

GOAL(S) FOR WORKOUT

TYPE OF RUN
- ○ LONG, SLOW DISTANCE RUN
- ○ SPEED/TRACK WORKOUT
- ○ MY REGULAR RUN

WHERE
- ○ INDOOR
- ○ OUTDOOR

ROUTE

DISTANCE

TIME OF DAY/NIGHT

TIME   **PACE**   **WEATHER**

EFFORT

| 1 EASY | 2 EASY+ | 3 OK! | 4 OOF | 5 OMG |

COMMENTS

FRIDAY

STRETCHING/WARM-UP

GOAL(S) FOR WORKOUT

TYPE OF RUN
- ○ LONG, SLOW DISTANCE RUN
- ○ SPEED/TRACK WORKOUT
- ○ MY REGULAR RUN

WHERE
- ○ INDOOR
- ○ OUTDOOR

ROUTE

DISTANCE

TIME OF DAY/NIGHT

TIME   **PACE**   **WEATHER**

EFFORT

| 1 EASY | 2 EASY+ | 3 OK! | 4 OOF | 5 OMG |

COMMENTS

SATURDAY

STRETCHING/WARM-UP

GOAL(S) FOR WORKOUT

TYPE OF RUN
- ○ LONG, SLOW DISTANCE RUN
- ○ SPEED/TRACK WORKOUT
- ○ MY REGULAR RUN

WHERE
- ○ INDOOR
- ○ OUTDOOR

ROUTE

DISTANCE

TIME OF DAY/NIGHT

TIME   **PACE**   **WEATHER**

EFFORT

| 1 EASY | 2 EASY+ | 3 OK! | 4 OOF | 5 OMG |

COMMENTS

SUNDAY

STRETCHING/WARM-UP

GOAL(S) FOR WORKOUT

TYPE OF RUN
- ○ LONG, SLOW DISTANCE RUN
- ○ SPEED/TRACK WORKOUT
- ○ MY REGULAR RUN

WHERE
- ○ INDOOR
- ○ OUTDOOR

ROUTE

DISTANCE

TIME OF DAY/NIGHT

TIME   **PACE**   **WEATHER**

EFFORT

| 1 EASY | 2 EASY+ | 3 OK! | 4 OOF | 5 OMG |

COMMENTS

WEEK 40

BEGIN DATE	END DATE

TOTAL MILEAGE THIS WEEK

MONDAY

STRETCHING/WARM-UP

GOAL(S) FOR WORKOUT

TYPE OF RUN
- ○ LONG, SLOW DISTANCE RUN
- ○ SPEED/TRACK WORKOUT
- ○ MY REGULAR RUN

WHERE
- ○ INDOOR
- ○ OUTDOOR

ROUTE

DISTANCE

TIME OF DAY/NIGHT

TIME   PACE   WEATHER

EFFORT

1 EASY	2 EASY+	3 OK!	4 OOF	5 OMG

COMMENTS

TUESDAY

STRETCHING/WARM-UP

GOAL(S) FOR WORKOUT

TYPE OF RUN
- ○ LONG, SLOW DISTANCE RUN
- ○ SPEED/TRACK WORKOUT
- ○ MY REGULAR RUN

WHERE
- ○ INDOOR
- ○ OUTDOOR

ROUTE

DISTANCE

TIME OF DAY/NIGHT

TIME   PACE   WEATHER

EFFORT

1 EASY	2 EASY+	3 OK!	4 OOF	5 OMG

COMMENTS

WEDNESDAY

STRETCHING/WARM-UP

GOAL(S) FOR WORKOUT

TYPE OF RUN
- ○ LONG, SLOW DISTANCE RUN
- ○ SPEED/TRACK WORKOUT
- ○ MY REGULAR RUN

WHERE
- ○ INDOOR
- ○ OUTDOOR

ROUTE

DISTANCE

TIME OF DAY/NIGHT

TIME   PACE   WEATHER

EFFORT

1 EASY	2 EASY+	3 OK!	4 OOF	5 OMG

COMMENTS

THURSDAY

STRETCHING/WARM-UP

GOAL(S) FOR WORKOUT

TYPE OF RUN
○ LONG, SLOW DISTANCE RUN
○ SPEED/TRACK WORKOUT
○ MY REGULAR RUN

WHERE
○ INDOOR
○ OUTDOOR

ROUTE

DISTANCE

TIME OF DAY/NIGHT

TIME   PACE   WEATHER

EFFORT
| 1 EASY | 2 EASY+ | 3 OK! | 4 OOF | 5 OMG |

COMMENTS

FRIDAY

STRETCHING/WARM-UP

GOAL(S) FOR WORKOUT

TYPE OF RUN
○ LONG, SLOW DISTANCE RUN
○ SPEED/TRACK WORKOUT
○ MY REGULAR RUN

WHERE
○ INDOOR
○ OUTDOOR

ROUTE

DISTANCE

TIME OF DAY/NIGHT

TIME   PACE   WEATHER

EFFORT
| 1 EASY | 2 EASY+ | 3 OK! | 4 OOF | 5 OMG |

COMMENTS

SATURDAY

STRETCHING/WARM-UP

GOAL(S) FOR WORKOUT

TYPE OF RUN
○ LONG, SLOW DISTANCE RUN
○ SPEED/TRACK WORKOUT
○ MY REGULAR RUN

WHERE
○ INDOOR
○ OUTDOOR

ROUTE

DISTANCE

TIME OF DAY/NIGHT

TIME   PACE   WEATHER

EFFORT
| 1 EASY | 2 EASY+ | 3 OK! | 4 OOF | 5 OMG |

COMMENTS

SUNDAY

STRETCHING/WARM-UP

GOAL(S) FOR WORKOUT

TYPE OF RUN
○ LONG, SLOW DISTANCE RUN
○ SPEED/TRACK WORKOUT
○ MY REGULAR RUN

WHERE
○ INDOOR
○ OUTDOOR

ROUTE

DISTANCE

TIME OF DAY/NIGHT

TIME   PACE   WEATHER

EFFORT
| 1 EASY | 2 EASY+ | 3 OK! | 4 OOF | 5 OMG |

COMMENTS

WEEK 41

BEGIN DATE

END DATE

TOTAL MILEAGE THIS WEEK

MONDAY

STRETCHING/WARM-UP

GOAL(S) FOR WORKOUT

TYPE OF RUN
- ○ LONG, SLOW DISTANCE RUN
- ○ SPEED/TRACK WORKOUT
- ○ MY REGULAR RUN

WHERE
- ○ INDOOR
- ○ OUTDOOR

ROUTE

DISTANCE

TIME OF DAY/NIGHT

TIME

PACE

WEATHER

EFFORT

| 1 EASY | 2 EASY+ | 3 OK! | 4 OOF | 5 OMG |

COMMENTS

TUESDAY

STRETCHING/WARM-UP

GOAL(S) FOR WORKOUT

TYPE OF RUN
- ○ LONG, SLOW DISTANCE RUN
- ○ SPEED/TRACK WORKOUT
- ○ MY REGULAR RUN

WHERE
- ○ INDOOR
- ○ OUTDOOR

ROUTE

DISTANCE

TIME OF DAY/NIGHT

TIME

PACE

WEATHER

EFFORT

| 1 EASY | 2 EASY+ | 3 OK! | 4 OOF | 5 OMG |

COMMENTS

WEDNESDAY

STRETCHING/WARM-UP

GOAL(S) FOR WORKOUT

TYPE OF RUN
- ○ LONG, SLOW DISTANCE RUN
- ○ SPEED/TRACK WORKOUT
- ○ MY REGULAR RUN

WHERE
- ○ INDOOR
- ○ OUTDOOR

ROUTE

DISTANCE

TIME OF DAY/NIGHT

TIME

PACE

WEATHER

EFFORT

| 1 EASY | 2 EASY+ | 3 OK! | 4 OOF | 5 OMG |

COMMENTS

THURSDAY

STRETCHING/WARM-UP

GOAL(S) FOR WORKOUT

TYPE OF RUN
- ○ LONG, SLOW DISTANCE RUN
- ○ SPEED/TRACK WORKOUT
- ○ MY REGULAR RUN

WHERE
- ○ INDOOR
- ○ OUTDOOR

ROUTE

DISTANCE

TIME OF DAY/NIGHT

TIME   PACE   WEATHER

EFFORT
| 1 EASY | 2 EASY+ | 3 OK! | 4 OOF | 5 OMG |

COMMENTS

FRIDAY

STRETCHING/WARM-UP

GOAL(S) FOR WORKOUT

TYPE OF RUN
- ○ LONG, SLOW DISTANCE RUN
- ○ SPEED/TRACK WORKOUT
- ○ MY REGULAR RUN

WHERE
- ○ INDOOR
- ○ OUTDOOR

ROUTE

DISTANCE

TIME OF DAY/NIGHT

TIME   PACE   WEATHER

EFFORT
| 1 EASY | 2 EASY+ | 3 OK! | 4 OOF | 5 OMG |

COMMENTS

SATURDAY

STRETCHING/WARM-UP

GOAL(S) FOR WORKOUT

TYPE OF RUN
- ○ LONG, SLOW DISTANCE RUN
- ○ SPEED/TRACK WORKOUT
- ○ MY REGULAR RUN

WHERE
- ○ INDOOR
- ○ OUTDOOR

ROUTE

DISTANCE

TIME OF DAY/NIGHT

TIME   PACE   WEATHER

EFFORT
| 1 EASY | 2 EASY+ | 3 OK! | 4 OOF | 5 OMG |

COMMENTS

SUNDAY

STRETCHING/WARM-UP

GOAL(S) FOR WORKOUT

TYPE OF RUN
- ○ LONG, SLOW DISTANCE RUN
- ○ SPEED/TRACK WORKOUT
- ○ MY REGULAR RUN

WHERE
- ○ INDOOR
- ○ OUTDOOR

ROUTE

DISTANCE

TIME OF DAY/NIGHT

TIME   PACE   WEATHER

EFFORT
| 1 EASY | 2 EASY+ | 3 OK! | 4 OOF | 5 OMG |

COMMENTS

WEEK 42

BEGIN DATE

END DATE

TOTAL MILEAGE THIS WEEK

MONDAY

STRETCHING/WARM-UP

GOAL(S) FOR WORKOUT

TYPE OF RUN
- ○ LONG, SLOW DISTANCE RUN
- ○ SPEED/TRACK WORKOUT
- ○ MY REGULAR RUN

WHERE
- ○ INDOOR
- ○ OUTDOOR

ROUTE

DISTANCE

TIME OF DAY/NIGHT

TIME   PACE   WEATHER

EFFORT

| 1 EASY | 2 EASY+ | 3 OK! | 4 OOF | 5 OMG |

COMMENTS

TUESDAY

STRETCHING/WARM-UP

GOAL(S) FOR WORKOUT

TYPE OF RUN
- ○ LONG, SLOW DISTANCE RUN
- ○ SPEED/TRACK WORKOUT
- ○ MY REGULAR RUN

WHERE
- ○ INDOOR
- ○ OUTDOOR

ROUTE

DISTANCE

TIME OF DAY/NIGHT

TIME   PACE   WEATHER

EFFORT

| 1 EASY | 2 EASY+ | 3 OK! | 4 OOF | 5 OMG |

COMMENTS

WEDNESDAY

STRETCHING/WARM-UP

GOAL(S) FOR WORKOUT

TYPE OF RUN
- ○ LONG, SLOW DISTANCE RUN
- ○ SPEED/TRACK WORKOUT
- ○ MY REGULAR RUN

WHERE
- ○ INDOOR
- ○ OUTDOOR

ROUTE

DISTANCE

TIME OF DAY/NIGHT

TIME   PACE   WEATHER

EFFORT

| 1 EASY | 2 EASY+ | 3 OK! | 4 OOF | 5 OMG |

COMMENTS

THURSDAY

STRETCHING/WARM-UP

GOAL(S) FOR WORKOUT

TYPE OF RUN
- ○ LONG, SLOW DISTANCE RUN
- ○ SPEED/TRACK WORKOUT
- ○ MY REGULAR RUN

WHERE
- ○ INDOOR
- ○ OUTDOOR

ROUTE

DISTANCE

TIME OF DAY/NIGHT

TIME   PACE   WEATHER

EFFORT

| 1 EASY | 2 EASY+ | 3 OK! | 4 OOF | 5 OMG |

COMMENTS

FRIDAY

STRETCHING/WARM-UP

GOAL(S) FOR WORKOUT

TYPE OF RUN
- ○ LONG, SLOW DISTANCE RUN
- ○ SPEED/TRACK WORKOUT
- ○ MY REGULAR RUN

WHERE
- ○ INDOOR
- ○ OUTDOOR

ROUTE

DISTANCE

TIME OF DAY/NIGHT

TIME   PACE   WEATHER

EFFORT

| 1 EASY | 2 EASY+ | 3 OK! | 4 OOF | 5 OMG |

COMMENTS

SATURDAY

STRETCHING/WARM-UP

GOAL(S) FOR WORKOUT

TYPE OF RUN
- ○ LONG, SLOW DISTANCE RUN
- ○ SPEED/TRACK WORKOUT
- ○ MY REGULAR RUN

WHERE
- ○ INDOOR
- ○ OUTDOOR

ROUTE

DISTANCE

TIME OF DAY/NIGHT

TIME   PACE   WEATHER

EFFORT

| 1 EASY | 2 EASY+ | 3 OK! | 4 OOF | 5 OMG |

COMMENTS

SUNDAY

STRETCHING/WARM-UP

GOAL(S) FOR WORKOUT

TYPE OF RUN
- ○ LONG, SLOW DISTANCE RUN
- ○ SPEED/TRACK WORKOUT
- ○ MY REGULAR RUN

WHERE
- ○ INDOOR
- ○ OUTDOOR

ROUTE

DISTANCE

TIME OF DAY/NIGHT

TIME   PACE   WEATHER

EFFORT

| 1 EASY | 2 EASY+ | 3 OK! | 4 OOF | 5 OMG |

COMMENTS

WEEK 43

BEGIN DATE	END DATE

TOTAL MILEAGE THIS WEEK

MONDAY

STRETCHING/WARM-UP

GOAL(S) FOR WORKOUT

TYPE OF RUN
- ○ LONG, SLOW DISTANCE RUN
- ○ SPEED/TRACK WORKOUT
- ○ MY REGULAR RUN

WHERE
- ○ INDOOR
- ○ OUTDOOR

ROUTE

DISTANCE

TIME OF DAY/NIGHT

TIME   PACE   WEATHER

EFFORT

| 1 EASY | 2 EASY+ | 3 OK! | 4 OOF | 5 OMG |

COMMENTS

TUESDAY

STRETCHING/WARM-UP

GOAL(S) FOR WORKOUT

TYPE OF RUN
- ○ LONG, SLOW DISTANCE RUN
- ○ SPEED/TRACK WORKOUT
- ○ MY REGULAR RUN

WHERE
- ○ INDOOR
- ○ OUTDOOR

ROUTE

DISTANCE

TIME OF DAY/NIGHT

TIME   PACE   WEATHER

EFFORT

| 1 EASY | 2 EASY+ | 3 OK! | 4 OOF | 5 OMG |

COMMENTS

WEDNESDAY

STRETCHING/WARM-UP

GOAL(S) FOR WORKOUT

TYPE OF RUN
- ○ LONG, SLOW DISTANCE RUN
- ○ SPEED/TRACK WORKOUT
- ○ MY REGULAR RUN

WHERE
- ○ INDOOR
- ○ OUTDOOR

ROUTE

DISTANCE

TIME OF DAY/NIGHT

TIME   PACE   WEATHER

EFFORT

| 1 EASY | 2 EASY+ | 3 OK! | 4 OOF | 5 OMG |

COMMENTS

THURSDAY

STRETCHING/WARM-UP

GOAL(S) FOR WORKOUT

TYPE OF RUN
- ○ LONG, SLOW DISTANCE RUN
- ○ SPEED/TRACK WORKOUT
- ○ MY REGULAR RUN

WHERE
- ○ INDOOR
- ○ OUTDOOR

ROUTE

DISTANCE

TIME OF DAY/NIGHT

TIME   **PACE**   **WEATHER**

EFFORT

| 1 EASY | 2 EASY+ | 3 OK! | 4 OOF | 5 OMG |

COMMENTS

FRIDAY

STRETCHING/WARM-UP

GOAL(S) FOR WORKOUT

TYPE OF RUN
- ○ LONG, SLOW DISTANCE RUN
- ○ SPEED/TRACK WORKOUT
- ○ MY REGULAR RUN

WHERE
- ○ INDOOR
- ○ OUTDOOR

ROUTE

DISTANCE

TIME OF DAY/NIGHT

TIME   **PACE**   **WEATHER**

EFFORT

| 1 EASY | 2 EASY+ | 3 OK! | 4 OOF | 5 OMG |

COMMENTS

SATURDAY

STRETCHING/WARM-UP

GOAL(S) FOR WORKOUT

TYPE OF RUN
- ○ LONG, SLOW DISTANCE RUN
- ○ SPEED/TRACK WORKOUT
- ○ MY REGULAR RUN

WHERE
- ○ INDOOR
- ○ OUTDOOR

ROUTE

DISTANCE

TIME OF DAY/NIGHT

TIME   **PACE**   **WEATHER**

EFFORT

| 1 EASY | 2 EASY+ | 3 OK! | 4 OOF | 5 OMG |

COMMENTS

SUNDAY

STRETCHING/WARM-UP

GOAL(S) FOR WORKOUT

TYPE OF RUN
- ○ LONG, SLOW DISTANCE RUN
- ○ SPEED/TRACK WORKOUT
- ○ MY REGULAR RUN

WHERE
- ○ INDOOR
- ○ OUTDOOR

ROUTE

DISTANCE

TIME OF DAY/NIGHT

TIME   **PACE**   **WEATHER**

EFFORT

| 1 EASY | 2 EASY+ | 3 OK! | 4 OOF | 5 OMG |

COMMENTS

MONDAY

STRETCHING/WARM-UP	DISTANCE		TIME OF DAY/NIGHT
GOAL(S) FOR WORKOUT	TIME	PACE	WEATHER

TYPE OF RUN
- ○ LONG, SLOW DISTANCE RUN
- ○ SPEED/TRACK WORKOUT
- ○ MY REGULAR RUN

WHERE
- ○ INDOOR
- ○ OUTDOOR

EFFORT   1 EASY   2 EASY+   3 OK!   4 OOF   5 OMG

COMMENTS

ROUTE

TUESDAY

STRETCHING/WARM-UP	DISTANCE		TIME OF DAY/NIGHT
GOAL(S) FOR WORKOUT	TIME	PACE	WEATHER

TYPE OF RUN
- ○ LONG, SLOW DISTANCE RUN
- ○ SPEED/TRACK WORKOUT
- ○ MY REGULAR RUN

WHERE
- ○ INDOOR
- ○ OUTDOOR

EFFORT   1 EASY   2 EASY+   3 OK!   4 OOF   5 OMG

COMMENTS

ROUTE

WEDNESDAY

STRETCHING/WARM-UP	DISTANCE		TIME OF DAY/NIGHT
GOAL(S) FOR WORKOUT	TIME	PACE	WEATHER

TYPE OF RUN
- ○ LONG, SLOW DISTANCE RUN
- ○ SPEED/TRACK WORKOUT
- ○ MY REGULAR RUN

WHERE
- ○ INDOOR
- ○ OUTDOOR

EFFORT   1 EASY   2 EASY+   3 OK!   4 OOF   5 OMG

COMMENTS

ROUTE

THURSDAY

STRETCHING/WARM-UP

GOAL(S) FOR WORKOUT

TYPE OF RUN
- ○ LONG, SLOW DISTANCE RUN
- ○ SPEED/TRACK WORKOUT
- ○ MY REGULAR RUN

WHERE
- ○ INDOOR
- ○ OUTDOOR

ROUTE

DISTANCE

TIME OF DAY/NIGHT

TIME **PACE** **WEATHER**

EFFORT

| 1 EASY | 2 EASY+ | 3 OK! | 4 OOF | 5 OMG |

COMMENTS

FRIDAY

STRETCHING/WARM-UP

GOAL(S) FOR WORKOUT

TYPE OF RUN
- ○ LONG, SLOW DISTANCE RUN
- ○ SPEED/TRACK WORKOUT
- ○ MY REGULAR RUN

WHERE
- ○ INDOOR
- ○ OUTDOOR

ROUTE

DISTANCE

TIME OF DAY/NIGHT

TIME **PACE** **WEATHER**

EFFORT

| 1 EASY | 2 EASY+ | 3 OK! | 4 OOF | 5 OMG |

COMMENTS

SATURDAY

STRETCHING/WARM-UP

GOAL(S) FOR WORKOUT

TYPE OF RUN
- ○ LONG, SLOW DISTANCE RUN
- ○ SPEED/TRACK WORKOUT
- ○ MY REGULAR RUN

WHERE
- ○ INDOOR
- ○ OUTDOOR

ROUTE

DISTANCE

TIME OF DAY/NIGHT

TIME **PACE** **WEATHER**

EFFORT

| 1 EASY | 2 EASY+ | 3 OK! | 4 OOF | 5 OMG |

COMMENTS

SUNDAY

STRETCHING/WARM-UP

GOAL(S) FOR WORKOUT

TYPE OF RUN
- ○ LONG, SLOW DISTANCE RUN
- ○ SPEED/TRACK WORKOUT
- ○ MY REGULAR RUN

WHERE
- ○ INDOOR
- ○ OUTDOOR

ROUTE

DISTANCE

TIME OF DAY/NIGHT

TIME **PACE** **WEATHER**

EFFORT

| 1 EASY | 2 EASY+ | 3 OK! | 4 OOF | 5 OMG |

COMMENTS

WEEK 45

BEGIN DATE	END DATE

TOTAL MILEAGE THIS WEEK

MONDAY

STRETCHING/WARM-UP	DISTANCE		TIME OF DAY/NIGHT

GOAL(S) FOR WORKOUT	TIME	PACE	WEATHER

TYPE OF RUN
- ○ LONG, SLOW DISTANCE RUN
- ○ SPEED/TRACK WORKOUT
- ○ MY REGULAR RUN

WHERE
- ○ INDOOR
- ○ OUTDOOR

EFFORT

1 EASY	2 EASY+	3 OK!	4 OOF	5 OMG

COMMENTS

ROUTE

TUESDAY

STRETCHING/WARM-UP	DISTANCE		TIME OF DAY/NIGHT

GOAL(S) FOR WORKOUT	TIME	PACE	WEATHER

TYPE OF RUN
- ○ LONG, SLOW DISTANCE RUN
- ○ SPEED/TRACK WORKOUT
- ○ MY REGULAR RUN

WHERE
- ○ INDOOR
- ○ OUTDOOR

EFFORT

1 EASY	2 EASY+	3 OK!	4 OOF	5 OMG

COMMENTS

ROUTE

WEDNESDAY

STRETCHING/WARM-UP	DISTANCE		TIME OF DAY/NIGHT

GOAL(S) FOR WORKOUT	TIME	PACE	WEATHER

TYPE OF RUN
- ○ LONG, SLOW DISTANCE RUN
- ○ SPEED/TRACK WORKOUT
- ○ MY REGULAR RUN

WHERE
- ○ INDOOR
- ○ OUTDOOR

EFFORT

1 EASY	2 EASY+	3 OK!	4 OOF	5 OMG

COMMENTS

ROUTE

THURSDAY

STRETCHING/WARM-UP

GOAL(S) FOR WORKOUT

TYPE OF RUN
- ○ LONG, SLOW DISTANCE RUN
- ○ SPEED/TRACK WORKOUT
- ○ MY REGULAR RUN

WHERE
- ○ INDOOR
- ○ OUTDOOR

ROUTE

DISTANCE

TIME OF DAY/NIGHT

TIME   PACE   WEATHER

EFFORT

| 1 EASY | 2 EASY+ | 3 OK! | 4 OOF | 5 OMG |

COMMENTS

FRIDAY

STRETCHING/WARM-UP

GOAL(S) FOR WORKOUT

TYPE OF RUN
- ○ LONG, SLOW DISTANCE RUN
- ○ SPEED/TRACK WORKOUT
- ○ MY REGULAR RUN

WHERE
- ○ INDOOR
- ○ OUTDOOR

ROUTE

DISTANCE

TIME OF DAY/NIGHT

TIME   PACE   WEATHER

EFFORT

| 1 EASY | 2 EASY+ | 3 OK! | 4 OOF | 5 OMG |

COMMENTS

SATURDAY

STRETCHING/WARM-UP

GOAL(S) FOR WORKOUT

TYPE OF RUN
- ○ LONG, SLOW DISTANCE RUN
- ○ SPEED/TRACK WORKOUT
- ○ MY REGULAR RUN

WHERE
- ○ INDOOR
- ○ OUTDOOR

ROUTE

DISTANCE

TIME OF DAY/NIGHT

TIME   PACE   WEATHER

EFFORT

| 1 EASY | 2 EASY+ | 3 OK! | 4 OOF | 5 OMG |

COMMENTS

SUNDAY

STRETCHING/WARM-UP

GOAL(S) FOR WORKOUT

TYPE OF RUN
- ○ LONG, SLOW DISTANCE RUN
- ○ SPEED/TRACK WORKOUT
- ○ MY REGULAR RUN

WHERE
- ○ INDOOR
- ○ OUTDOOR

ROUTE

DISTANCE

TIME OF DAY/NIGHT

TIME   PACE   WEATHER

EFFORT

| 1 EASY | 2 EASY+ | 3 OK! | 4 OOF | 5 OMG |

COMMENTS

MONDAY

STRETCHING/WARM-UP

GOAL(S) FOR WORKOUT

TYPE OF RUN
- ○ LONG, SLOW DISTANCE RUN
- ○ SPEED/TRACK WORKOUT
- ○ MY REGULAR RUN

WHERE
- ○ INDOOR
- ○ OUTDOOR

ROUTE

DISTANCE

TIME OF DAY/NIGHT

TIME   PACE   WEATHER

EFFORT

| 1 EASY | 2 EASY+ | 3 OK! | 4 OOF | 5 OMG |

COMMENTS

TUESDAY

STRETCHING/WARM-UP

GOAL(S) FOR WORKOUT

TYPE OF RUN
- ○ LONG, SLOW DISTANCE RUN
- ○ SPEED/TRACK WORKOUT
- ○ MY REGULAR RUN

WHERE
- ○ INDOOR
- ○ OUTDOOR

ROUTE

DISTANCE

TIME OF DAY/NIGHT

TIME   PACE   WEATHER

EFFORT

| 1 EASY | 2 EASY+ | 3 OK! | 4 OOF | 5 OMG |

COMMENTS

WEDNESDAY

STRETCHING/WARM-UP

GOAL(S) FOR WORKOUT

TYPE OF RUN
- ○ LONG, SLOW DISTANCE RUN
- ○ SPEED/TRACK WORKOUT
- ○ MY REGULAR RUN

WHERE
- ○ INDOOR
- ○ OUTDOOR

ROUTE

DISTANCE

TIME OF DAY/NIGHT

TIME   PACE   WEATHER

EFFORT

| 1 EASY | 2 EASY+ | 3 OK! | 4 OOF | 5 OMG |

COMMENTS

THURSDAY

STRETCHING/WARM-UP

GOAL(S) FOR WORKOUT

TYPE OF RUN
○ LONG, SLOW DISTANCE RUN
○ SPEED/TRACK WORKOUT
○ MY REGULAR RUN

WHERE
○ INDOOR
○ OUTDOOR

ROUTE

DISTANCE

TIME OF DAY/NIGHT

TIME

PACE

WEATHER

EFFORT

| 1 EASY | 2 EASY+ | 3 OK! | 4 OOF | 5 OMG |

COMMENTS

FRIDAY

STRETCHING/WARM-UP

GOAL(S) FOR WORKOUT

TYPE OF RUN
○ LONG, SLOW DISTANCE RUN
○ SPEED/TRACK WORKOUT
○ MY REGULAR RUN

WHERE
○ INDOOR
○ OUTDOOR

ROUTE

DISTANCE

TIME OF DAY/NIGHT

TIME

PACE

WEATHER

EFFORT

| 1 EASY | 2 EASY+ | 3 OK! | 4 OOF | 5 OMG |

COMMENTS

SATURDAY

STRETCHING/WARM-UP

GOAL(S) FOR WORKOUT

TYPE OF RUN
○ LONG, SLOW DISTANCE RUN
○ SPEED/TRACK WORKOUT
○ MY REGULAR RUN

WHERE
○ INDOOR
○ OUTDOOR

ROUTE

DISTANCE

TIME OF DAY/NIGHT

TIME

PACE

WEATHER

EFFORT

| 1 EASY | 2 EASY+ | 3 OK! | 4 OOF | 5 OMG |

COMMENTS

SUNDAY

STRETCHING/WARM-UP

GOAL(S) FOR WORKOUT

TYPE OF RUN
○ LONG, SLOW DISTANCE RUN
○ SPEED/TRACK WORKOUT
○ MY REGULAR RUN

WHERE
○ INDOOR
○ OUTDOOR

ROUTE

DISTANCE

TIME OF DAY/NIGHT

TIME

PACE

WEATHER

EFFORT

| 1 EASY | 2 EASY+ | 3 OK! | 4 OOF | 5 OMG |

COMMENTS

WEEK 47

BEGIN DATE

END DATE

TOTAL MILEAGE THIS WEEK

MONDAY

STRETCHING/WARM-UP

DISTANCE

TIME OF DAY/NIGHT

GOAL(S) FOR WORKOUT

TIME

PACE

WEATHER

TYPE OF RUN
- LONG, SLOW DISTANCE RUN
- SPEED/TRACK WORKOUT
- MY REGULAR RUN

WHERE
- INDOOR
- OUTDOOR

EFFORT

| 1 EASY | 2 EASY+ | 3 OK! | 4 OOF | 5 OMG |

COMMENTS

ROUTE

TUESDAY

STRETCHING/WARM-UP

DISTANCE

TIME OF DAY/NIGHT

GOAL(S) FOR WORKOUT

TIME

PACE

WEATHER

TYPE OF RUN
- LONG, SLOW DISTANCE RUN
- SPEED/TRACK WORKOUT
- MY REGULAR RUN

WHERE
- INDOOR
- OUTDOOR

EFFORT

| 1 EASY | 2 EASY+ | 3 OK! | 4 OOF | 5 OMG |

COMMENTS

ROUTE

WEDNESDAY

STRETCHING/WARM-UP

DISTANCE

TIME OF DAY/NIGHT

GOAL(S) FOR WORKOUT

TIME

PACE

WEATHER

TYPE OF RUN
- LONG, SLOW DISTANCE RUN
- SPEED/TRACK WORKOUT
- MY REGULAR RUN

WHERE
- INDOOR
- OUTDOOR

EFFORT

| 1 EASY | 2 EASY+ | 3 OK! | 4 OOF | 5 OMG |

COMMENTS

ROUTE

THURSDAY

STRETCHING/WARM-UP

GOAL(S) FOR WORKOUT

TYPE OF RUN
○ LONG, SLOW DISTANCE RUN
○ SPEED/TRACK WORKOUT
○ MY REGULAR RUN

WHERE
○ INDOOR
○ OUTDOOR

ROUTE

DISTANCE

TIME OF DAY/NIGHT

TIME   PACE   WEATHER

EFFORT | 1 EASY | 2 EASY+ | 3 OK! | 4 OOF | 5 OMG |

COMMENTS

FRIDAY

STRETCHING/WARM-UP

GOAL(S) FOR WORKOUT

TYPE OF RUN
○ LONG, SLOW DISTANCE RUN
○ SPEED/TRACK WORKOUT
○ MY REGULAR RUN

WHERE
○ INDOOR
○ OUTDOOR

ROUTE

DISTANCE

TIME OF DAY/NIGHT

TIME   PACE   WEATHER

EFFORT | 1 EASY | 2 EASY+ | 3 OK! | 4 OOF | 5 OMG |

COMMENTS

SATURDAY

STRETCHING/WARM-UP

GOAL(S) FOR WORKOUT

TYPE OF RUN
○ LONG, SLOW DISTANCE RUN
○ SPEED/TRACK WORKOUT
○ MY REGULAR RUN

WHERE
○ INDOOR
○ OUTDOOR

ROUTE

DISTANCE

TIME OF DAY/NIGHT

TIME   PACE   WEATHER

EFFORT | 1 EASY | 2 EASY+ | 3 OK! | 4 OOF | 5 OMG |

COMMENTS

SUNDAY

STRETCHING/WARM-UP

GOAL(S) FOR WORKOUT

TYPE OF RUN
○ LONG, SLOW DISTANCE RUN
○ SPEED/TRACK WORKOUT
○ MY REGULAR RUN

WHERE
○ INDOOR
○ OUTDOOR

ROUTE

DISTANCE

TIME OF DAY/NIGHT

TIME   PACE   WEATHER

EFFORT | 1 EASY | 2 EASY+ | 3 OK! | 4 OOF | 5 OMG |

COMMENTS

WEEK 48

BEGIN DATE

END DATE

TOTAL MILEAGE THIS WEEK

MONDAY

STRETCHING/WARM-UP

GOAL(S) FOR WORKOUT

TYPE OF RUN
- ○ LONG, SLOW DISTANCE RUN
- ○ SPEED/TRACK WORKOUT
- ○ MY REGULAR RUN

WHERE
- ○ INDOOR
- ○ OUTDOOR

ROUTE

DISTANCE

TIME OF DAY/NIGHT

TIME

PACE

WEATHER

EFFORT

| 1 EASY | 2 EASY+ | 3 OK! | 4 OOF | 5 OMG |

COMMENTS

TUESDAY

STRETCHING/WARM-UP

GOAL(S) FOR WORKOUT

TYPE OF RUN
- ○ LONG, SLOW DISTANCE RUN
- ○ SPEED/TRACK WORKOUT
- ○ MY REGULAR RUN

WHERE
- ○ INDOOR
- ○ OUTDOOR

ROUTE

DISTANCE

TIME OF DAY/NIGHT

TIME

PACE

WEATHER

EFFORT

| 1 EASY | 2 EASY+ | 3 OK! | 4 OOF | 5 OMG |

COMMENTS

WEDNESDAY

STRETCHING/WARM-UP

GOAL(S) FOR WORKOUT

TYPE OF RUN
- ○ LONG, SLOW DISTANCE RUN
- ○ SPEED/TRACK WORKOUT
- ○ MY REGULAR RUN

WHERE
- ○ INDOOR
- ○ OUTDOOR

ROUTE

DISTANCE

TIME OF DAY/NIGHT

TIME

PACE

WEATHER

EFFORT

| 1 EASY | 2 EASY+ | 3 OK! | 4 OOF | 5 OMG |

COMMENTS

THURSDAY

STRETCHING/WARM-UP

GOAL(S) FOR WORKOUT

TYPE OF RUN
- ○ LONG, SLOW DISTANCE RUN
- ○ SPEED/TRACK WORKOUT
- ○ MY REGULAR RUN

WHERE
- ○ INDOOR
- ○ OUTDOOR

ROUTE

DISTANCE

TIME OF DAY/NIGHT

TIME **PACE** **WEATHER**

EFFORT

| 1 EASY | 2 EASY+ | 3 OK! | 4 OOF | 5 OMG |

COMMENTS

FRIDAY

STRETCHING/WARM-UP

GOAL(S) FOR WORKOUT

TYPE OF RUN
- ○ LONG, SLOW DISTANCE RUN
- ○ SPEED/TRACK WORKOUT
- ○ MY REGULAR RUN

WHERE
- ○ INDOOR
- ○ OUTDOOR

ROUTE

DISTANCE

TIME OF DAY/NIGHT

TIME **PACE** **WEATHER**

EFFORT

| 1 EASY | 2 EASY+ | 3 OK! | 4 OOF | 5 OMG |

COMMENTS

SATURDAY

STRETCHING/WARM-UP

GOAL(S) FOR WORKOUT

TYPE OF RUN
- ○ LONG, SLOW DISTANCE RUN
- ○ SPEED/TRACK WORKOUT
- ○ MY REGULAR RUN

WHERE
- ○ INDOOR
- ○ OUTDOOR

ROUTE

DISTANCE

TIME OF DAY/NIGHT

TIME **PACE** **WEATHER**

EFFORT

| 1 EASY | 2 EASY+ | 3 OK! | 4 OOF | 5 OMG |

COMMENTS

SUNDAY

STRETCHING/WARM-UP

GOAL(S) FOR WORKOUT

TYPE OF RUN
- ○ LONG, SLOW DISTANCE RUN
- ○ SPEED/TRACK WORKOUT
- ○ MY REGULAR RUN

WHERE
- ○ INDOOR
- ○ OUTDOOR

ROUTE

DISTANCE

TIME OF DAY/NIGHT

TIME **PACE** **WEATHER**

EFFORT

| 1 EASY | 2 EASY+ | 3 OK! | 4 OOF | 5 OMG |

COMMENTS

WEEK 49

BEGIN DATE

END DATE

TOTAL MILEAGE THIS WEEK

MONDAY

STRETCHING/WARM-UP

DISTANCE

TIME OF DAY/NIGHT

GOAL(S) FOR WORKOUT

TIME

PACE

WEATHER

TYPE OF RUN
- LONG, SLOW DISTANCE RUN
- SPEED/TRACK WORKOUT
- MY REGULAR RUN

WHERE
- INDOOR
- OUTDOOR

EFFORT

| 1 EASY | 2 EASY+ | 3 OK! | 4 OOF | 5 OMG |

COMMENTS

ROUTE

TUESDAY

STRETCHING/WARM-UP

DISTANCE

TIME OF DAY/NIGHT

GOAL(S) FOR WORKOUT

TIME

PACE

WEATHER

TYPE OF RUN
- LONG, SLOW DISTANCE RUN
- SPEED/TRACK WORKOUT
- MY REGULAR RUN

WHERE
- INDOOR
- OUTDOOR

EFFORT

| 1 EASY | 2 EASY+ | 3 OK! | 4 OOF | 5 OMG |

COMMENTS

ROUTE

WEDNESDAY

STRETCHING/WARM-UP

DISTANCE

TIME OF DAY/NIGHT

GOAL(S) FOR WORKOUT

TIME

PACE

WEATHER

TYPE OF RUN
- LONG, SLOW DISTANCE RUN
- SPEED/TRACK WORKOUT
- MY REGULAR RUN

WHERE
- INDOOR
- OUTDOOR

EFFORT

| 1 EASY | 2 EASY+ | 3 OK! | 4 OOF | 5 OMG |

COMMENTS

ROUTE

THURSDAY

STRETCHING/WARM-UP

GOAL(S) FOR WORKOUT

TYPE OF RUN
- ○ LONG, SLOW DISTANCE RUN
- ○ SPEED/TRACK WORKOUT
- ○ MY REGULAR RUN

WHERE
- ○ INDOOR
- ○ OUTDOOR

ROUTE

DISTANCE

TIME OF DAY/NIGHT

TIME **PACE** **WEATHER**

EFFORT
| 1 EASY | 2 EASY+ | 3 OK! | 4 OOF | 5 OMG |

COMMENTS

FRIDAY

STRETCHING/WARM-UP

GOAL(S) FOR WORKOUT

TYPE OF RUN
- ○ LONG, SLOW DISTANCE RUN
- ○ SPEED/TRACK WORKOUT
- ○ MY REGULAR RUN

WHERE
- ○ INDOOR
- ○ OUTDOOR

ROUTE

DISTANCE

TIME OF DAY/NIGHT

TIME **PACE** **WEATHER**

EFFORT
| 1 EASY | 2 EASY+ | 3 OK! | 4 OOF | 5 OMG |

COMMENTS

SATURDAY

STRETCHING/WARM-UP

GOAL(S) FOR WORKOUT

TYPE OF RUN
- ○ LONG, SLOW DISTANCE RUN
- ○ SPEED/TRACK WORKOUT
- ○ MY REGULAR RUN

WHERE
- ○ INDOOR
- ○ OUTDOOR

ROUTE

DISTANCE

TIME OF DAY/NIGHT

TIME **PACE** **WEATHER**

EFFORT
| 1 EASY | 2 EASY+ | 3 OK! | 4 OOF | 5 OMG |

COMMENTS

SUNDAY

STRETCHING/WARM-UP

GOAL(S) FOR WORKOUT

TYPE OF RUN
- ○ LONG, SLOW DISTANCE RUN
- ○ SPEED/TRACK WORKOUT
- ○ MY REGULAR RUN

WHERE
- ○ INDOOR
- ○ OUTDOOR

ROUTE

DISTANCE

TIME OF DAY/NIGHT

TIME **PACE** **WEATHER**

EFFORT
| 1 EASY | 2 EASY+ | 3 OK! | 4 OOF | 5 OMG |

COMMENTS

WEEK 50

BEGIN DATE

END DATE

TOTAL MILEAGE THIS WEEK

MONDAY

STRETCHING/WARM-UP

GOAL(S) FOR WORKOUT

TYPE OF RUN
- ○ LONG, SLOW DISTANCE RUN
- ○ SPEED/TRACK WORKOUT
- ○ MY REGULAR RUN

WHERE
- ○ INDOOR
- ○ OUTDOOR

ROUTE

DISTANCE

TIME OF DAY/NIGHT

TIME   PACE   WEATHER

EFFORT
| 1 EASY | 2 EASY+ | 3 OK! | 4 OOF | 5 OMG |

COMMENTS

TUESDAY

STRETCHING/WARM-UP

GOAL(S) FOR WORKOUT

TYPE OF RUN
- ○ LONG, SLOW DISTANCE RUN
- ○ SPEED/TRACK WORKOUT
- ○ MY REGULAR RUN

WHERE
- ○ INDOOR
- ○ OUTDOOR

ROUTE

DISTANCE

TIME OF DAY/NIGHT

TIME   PACE   WEATHER

EFFORT
| 1 EASY | 2 EASY+ | 3 OK! | 4 OOF | 5 OMG |

COMMENTS

WEDNESDAY

STRETCHING/WARM-UP

GOAL(S) FOR WORKOUT

TYPE OF RUN
- ○ LONG, SLOW DISTANCE RUN
- ○ SPEED/TRACK WORKOUT
- ○ MY REGULAR RUN

WHERE
- ○ INDOOR
- ○ OUTDOOR

ROUTE

DISTANCE

TIME OF DAY/NIGHT

TIME   PACE   WEATHER

EFFORT
| 1 EASY | 2 EASY+ | 3 OK! | 4 OOF | 5 OMG |

COMMENTS

THURSDAY

STRETCHING/WARM-UP

GOAL(S) FOR WORKOUT

TYPE OF RUN
○ LONG, SLOW DISTANCE RUN
○ SPEED/TRACK WORKOUT
○ MY REGULAR RUN

WHERE
○ INDOOR
○ OUTDOOR

ROUTE

DISTANCE

TIME OF DAY/NIGHT

TIME

PACE

WEATHER

EFFORT

| 1 EASY | 2 EASY+ | 3 OK! | 4 OOF | 5 OMG |

COMMENTS

FRIDAY

STRETCHING/WARM-UP

GOAL(S) FOR WORKOUT

TYPE OF RUN
○ LONG, SLOW DISTANCE RUN
○ SPEED/TRACK WORKOUT
○ MY REGULAR RUN

WHERE
○ INDOOR
○ OUTDOOR

ROUTE

DISTANCE

TIME OF DAY/NIGHT

TIME

PACE

WEATHER

EFFORT

| 1 EASY | 2 EASY+ | 3 OK! | 4 OOF | 5 OMG |

COMMENTS

SATURDAY

STRETCHING/WARM-UP

GOAL(S) FOR WORKOUT

TYPE OF RUN
○ LONG, SLOW DISTANCE RUN
○ SPEED/TRACK WORKOUT
○ MY REGULAR RUN

WHERE
○ INDOOR
○ OUTDOOR

ROUTE

DISTANCE

TIME OF DAY/NIGHT

TIME

PACE

WEATHER

EFFORT

| 1 EASY | 2 EASY+ | 3 OK! | 4 OOF | 5 OMG |

COMMENTS

SUNDAY

STRETCHING/WARM-UP

GOAL(S) FOR WORKOUT

TYPE OF RUN
○ LONG, SLOW DISTANCE RUN
○ SPEED/TRACK WORKOUT
○ MY REGULAR RUN

WHERE
○ INDOOR
○ OUTDOOR

ROUTE

DISTANCE

TIME OF DAY/NIGHT

TIME

PACE

WEATHER

EFFORT

| 1 EASY | 2 EASY+ | 3 OK! | 4 OOF | 5 OMG |

COMMENTS

WEEK 51

BEGIN DATE

END DATE

TOTAL MILEAGE THIS WEEK

MONDAY

STRETCHING/WARM-UP

DISTANCE

TIME OF DAY/NIGHT

GOAL(S) FOR WORKOUT

TIME

PACE

WEATHER

TYPE OF RUN
- ○ LONG, SLOW DISTANCE RUN
- ○ SPEED/TRACK WORKOUT
- ○ MY REGULAR RUN

WHERE
- ○ INDOOR
- ○ OUTDOOR

EFFORT

| 1 EASY | 2 EASY+ | 3 OK! | 4 OOF | 5 OMG |

COMMENTS

ROUTE

TUESDAY

STRETCHING/WARM-UP

DISTANCE

TIME OF DAY/NIGHT

GOAL(S) FOR WORKOUT

TIME

PACE

WEATHER

TYPE OF RUN
- ○ LONG, SLOW DISTANCE RUN
- ○ SPEED/TRACK WORKOUT
- ○ MY REGULAR RUN

WHERE
- ○ INDOOR
- ○ OUTDOOR

EFFORT

| 1 EASY | 2 EASY+ | 3 OK! | 4 OOF | 5 OMG |

COMMENTS

ROUTE

WEDNESDAY

STRETCHING/WARM-UP

DISTANCE

TIME OF DAY/NIGHT

GOAL(S) FOR WORKOUT

TIME

PACE

WEATHER

TYPE OF RUN
- ○ LONG, SLOW DISTANCE RUN
- ○ SPEED/TRACK WORKOUT
- ○ MY REGULAR RUN

WHERE
- ○ INDOOR
- ○ OUTDOOR

EFFORT

| 1 EASY | 2 EASY+ | 3 OK! | 4 OOF | 5 OMG |

COMMENTS

ROUTE

THURSDAY

STRETCHING/WARM-UP

GOAL(S) FOR WORKOUT

TYPE OF RUN
- ○ LONG, SLOW DISTANCE RUN
- ○ SPEED/TRACK WORKOUT
- ○ MY REGULAR RUN

WHERE
- ○ INDOOR
- ○ OUTDOOR

ROUTE

DISTANCE

TIME OF DAY/NIGHT

TIME   **PACE**   **WEATHER**

EFFORT

1	2	3	4	5
EASY	EASY+	OK!	OOF	OMG

COMMENTS

FRIDAY

STRETCHING/WARM-UP

GOAL(S) FOR WORKOUT

TYPE OF RUN
- ○ LONG, SLOW DISTANCE RUN
- ○ SPEED/TRACK WORKOUT
- ○ MY REGULAR RUN

WHERE
- ○ INDOOR
- ○ OUTDOOR

ROUTE

DISTANCE

TIME OF DAY/NIGHT

TIME   **PACE**   **WEATHER**

EFFORT

1	2	3	4	5
EASY	EASY+	OK!	OOF	OMG

COMMENTS

SATURDAY

STRETCHING/WARM-UP

GOAL(S) FOR WORKOUT

TYPE OF RUN
- ○ LONG, SLOW DISTANCE RUN
- ○ SPEED/TRACK WORKOUT
- ○ MY REGULAR RUN

WHERE
- ○ INDOOR
- ○ OUTDOOR

ROUTE

DISTANCE

TIME OF DAY/NIGHT

TIME   **PACE**   **WEATHER**

EFFORT

1	2	3	4	5
EASY	EASY+	OK!	OOF	OMG

COMMENTS

SUNDAY

STRETCHING/WARM-UP

GOAL(S) FOR WORKOUT

TYPE OF RUN
- ○ LONG, SLOW DISTANCE RUN
- ○ SPEED/TRACK WORKOUT
- ○ MY REGULAR RUN

WHERE
- ○ INDOOR
- ○ OUTDOOR

ROUTE

DISTANCE

TIME OF DAY/NIGHT

TIME   **PACE**   **WEATHER**

EFFORT

1	2	3	4	5
EASY	EASY+	OK!	OOF	OMG

COMMENTS

WEEK 52

BEGIN DATE

END DATE

TOTAL MILEAGE THIS WEEK

MONDAY

STRETCHING/WARM-UP

GOAL(S) FOR WORKOUT

TYPE OF RUN
- ○ LONG, SLOW DISTANCE RUN
- ○ SPEED/TRACK WORKOUT
- ○ MY REGULAR RUN

WHERE
- ○ INDOOR
- ○ OUTDOOR

ROUTE

DISTANCE

TIME OF DAY/NIGHT

TIME

PACE

WEATHER

EFFORT

| 1 EASY | 2 EASY+ | 3 OK! | 4 OOF | 5 OMG |

COMMENTS

TUESDAY

STRETCHING/WARM-UP

GOAL(S) FOR WORKOUT

TYPE OF RUN
- ○ LONG, SLOW DISTANCE RUN
- ○ SPEED/TRACK WORKOUT
- ○ MY REGULAR RUN

WHERE
- ○ INDOOR
- ○ OUTDOOR

ROUTE

DISTANCE

TIME OF DAY/NIGHT

TIME

PACE

WEATHER

EFFORT

| 1 EASY | 2 EASY+ | 3 OK! | 4 OOF | 5 OMG |

COMMENTS

WEDNESDAY

STRETCHING/WARM-UP

GOAL(S) FOR WORKOUT

TYPE OF RUN
- ○ LONG, SLOW DISTANCE RUN
- ○ SPEED/TRACK WORKOUT
- ○ MY REGULAR RUN

WHERE
- ○ INDOOR
- ○ OUTDOOR

ROUTE

DISTANCE

TIME OF DAY/NIGHT

TIME

PACE

WEATHER

EFFORT

| 1 EASY | 2 EASY+ | 3 OK! | 4 OOF | 5 OMG |

COMMENTS

THURSDAY

STRETCHING/WARM-UP

GOAL(S) FOR WORKOUT

TYPE OF RUN
- ○ LONG, SLOW DISTANCE RUN
- ○ SPEED/TRACK WORKOUT
- ○ MY REGULAR RUN

WHERE
- ○ INDOOR
- ○ OUTDOOR

ROUTE

DISTANCE

TIME OF DAY/NIGHT

TIME   PACE   WEATHER

EFFORT
| 1 EASY | 2 EASY+ | 3 OK! | 4 OOF | 5 OMG |

COMMENTS

FRIDAY

STRETCHING/WARM-UP

GOAL(S) FOR WORKOUT

TYPE OF RUN
- ○ LONG, SLOW DISTANCE RUN
- ○ SPEED/TRACK WORKOUT
- ○ MY REGULAR RUN

WHERE
- ○ INDOOR
- ○ OUTDOOR

ROUTE

DISTANCE

TIME OF DAY/NIGHT

TIME   PACE   WEATHER

EFFORT
| 1 EASY | 2 EASY+ | 3 OK! | 4 OOF | 5 OMG |

COMMENTS

SATURDAY

STRETCHING/WARM-UP

GOAL(S) FOR WORKOUT

TYPE OF RUN
- ○ LONG, SLOW DISTANCE RUN
- ○ SPEED/TRACK WORKOUT
- ○ MY REGULAR RUN

WHERE
- ○ INDOOR
- ○ OUTDOOR

ROUTE

DISTANCE

TIME OF DAY/NIGHT

TIME   PACE   WEATHER

EFFORT
| 1 EASY | 2 EASY+ | 3 OK! | 4 OOF | 5 OMG |

COMMENTS

SUNDAY

STRETCHING/WARM-UP

GOAL(S) FOR WORKOUT

TYPE OF RUN
- ○ LONG, SLOW DISTANCE RUN
- ○ SPEED/TRACK WORKOUT
- ○ MY REGULAR RUN

WHERE
- ○ INDOOR
- ○ OUTDOOR

ROUTE

DISTANCE

TIME OF DAY/NIGHT

TIME   PACE   WEATHER

EFFORT
| 1 EASY | 2 EASY+ | 3 OK! | 4 OOF | 5 OMG |

COMMENTS

NOTES

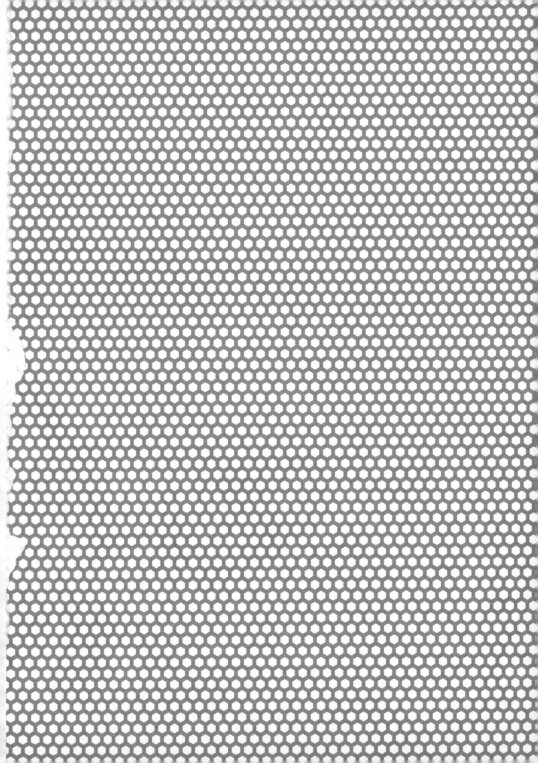